AF696633

BETTER *Blood Pressure*

First published in 1991 by
Sally Milner Publishing Pty Ltd
17 Wharf Road
Birchgrove NSW 2041 Australia

© Rob Edwards

Production by Sylvana Scannapiego,
Island Graphics
Design by Doric Order
Cartoons by John Kinnear
Accessories by Dean Saunders
Typeset in Australia by Asset Typesetting Pty Ltd
Printed in Australia by The Book Printer

National Library of Australia
Cataloguing-in-Publication data:

Edwards, Rob (Rob John)
Better Blood pressure.

ISBN 1 86351 030 3.

1. Hypertension – Popular works. I. Title.

616.13206

All rights reserved. No part of this publication may be reproduced, stored in a retrieval system or transmitted in any form or by any means, electronic, mechanical, photocopying, recording or otherwise, without prior written permission of the copyright holders.

Distributed in Australia by Transworld Publishers

Cover: *Foxglove* 1986/87
Lesley Dumbrell
acrylic on canvas (detail)
Collection of the Art Gallery of Western Australia, Perth.
Represented by Christine Abrahams Gallery, Melbourne.

BETTER Blood Pressure

A NEW PROGRAM TO RELIEVE HYPERTENSION

ROB EDWARDS

SALLY MILNER PUBLISHING

DEDICATED TO MY WIFE AND MY FATHER:

Annette thank you for your love and support while I've been chasing my dreams. Also for sharing with me our two beautiful girls.

Dad, thank you for the words —

'If you're going to do a job — take your time and do it properly.'

As a kid I listened to the words.
As a man I try to live by them.

READER'S FEEDBACK WELCOMED

The author invites comments, suggestions and inquiries. Please address correspondence to Harry and Rob, P.O. Box E12, Corrimal East NSW 2518.

Contents

Acknowledgements *vi*

Forewords *vii*

Introduction *1*

Your Aim *4*

Hypertension: What Does It Mean? *7*

The Excessive 'S's: Be A Winner *12*

How It All Works *21*

Doctor's Information Sheet *30*

Weigh Less *31*

Good Eating Guidelines *38*

Increase Activity *56*

Not Too Much Grog *64*

No More Smokes *70*

Ease Back On Salt *74*

Relax *78*

Harry's Healthy Hints and Recipes *86*

Record Section *114*

Acknowledgements

John Kinnear (Cartoon characters), a multi-talented art director and co-founder of Dingo Rock Graphic Design Studios. (042) 85 2802.

Dean Saunders (Accessories), at the age of 15 (1990) Dean's talent is sure to take him a long way in the art industry.

A special thank you to **Robyn Jarvis** for your assistance in developing the Good Eating Guidelines and your support in general.

Thanks also to:

Robyn Bornhorst and Margaret Bornhorst-Kairies for reviewing the original manuscript and encouragement. Also Margaret for your assistance in developing the Stress Rating Questionnaire.

Carmel Bellette for typing the original manuscript.

Marie Edwards and Cecilia Barker for your tremendous support and interesting challenges in the health field.

Ian Mackie, Laurie Axford and Ruth Odins for your great ability to communicate the principles of good health. I have learned from your example.

The clients of the Axford Jones Centre (Cronulla) who have achieved so much in terms of their personal health. You are a great inspiration to any health professional.

Julie Denman for your interest and support. It's a delight when a client becomes a friend.

Barbara Mobbs for your valuable assistance in steering this book along the path that it has taken.

Doug Malouf — yes Doug, I'm keeping it simple.

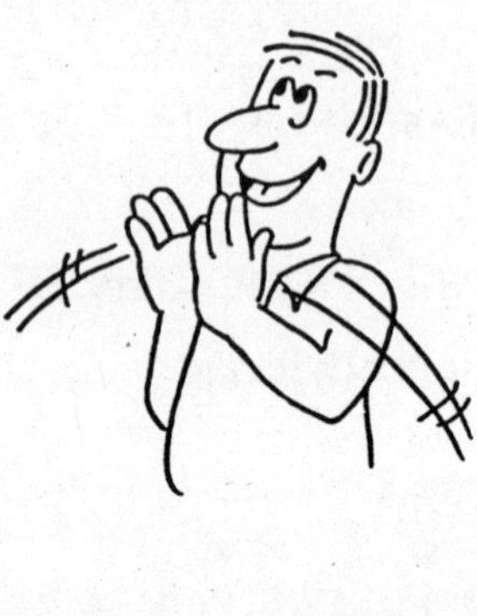

FOREWORD BY ROBYN WILLIAMS

My first mistake was choosing the wrong parents. On being told that, my inclination was to demand, 'So what am I supposed to do? Get born again biologically'?

But it's remarkable how set one's genes can be. On a recent trip back to Wales I saw my little sister (well, she's ten years younger than I am), whom I hadn't talked to for close to a decade. After the family gossip came the medical report. Her blood pressure symptoms turn out to be precisely the same as mine. Our brother, whom I'd also not seen in years, also matches me exactly. 'It's like a bloody computer program' we agreed.

My second mistake had been to dismiss the problem as commonplace. I'd been diagnosed as hypertensive in 1980, as so often happens, during a routine medical inspection for insurance purposes. Knowing that one-fifth of Australians will register suspect pressures, it's easy to seek safety in numbers. But then, after only a couple of months delaying, I applied retaliatory measures. I ran *every day.* Salt was banned. My blood pressure plummetted from a worrying 150/100 to a comfortable 120/70.

During the last ten years, though, as the body adjusts to the emergency remedies you apply (weight is lost quickly as you begin an exercise regime, then creeps back up as muscle and recidivism form), it became clear that a broader attack is needed. And the delightful discovery is that it all involves measures that are worthwhile anyway.

I resisted drugs, mainly because it seemed to imply a loss of control. But they have their place, especially the modern ones, which can be so well suited to a particular person. Nothing, however, can be more appropriate than the self-help routine that Rob Edwards has arranged in this book. It gives you reachable targets and amusing explanations. So good, in fact, that someone whose blood pressure is untroubled could well be advised to adopt most of the measures in any case. The dietary, exercise and non-smoking advice is impeccable.

As for the Alcohol Free Days, well, I'm working up to one of those. Stand by for miracles!

Robyn Williams

FOREWORD BY PROFESSOR W. A. LITTLER

Hypertension (high blood pressure) is a common finding in developed societies and a major cause of ill health and premature death. Indeed the risk of death and cardiovascular disease is closely linked to blood pressure levels; the higher the pressure, the greater the risk.

The consequences of hypertension are potentially correctable by lowering the blood pressure. Over the past 30 years we have witnessed the development and use of an increasing list of potent hypotensive drugs with increasingly less troublesome side effects. Such drugs can lull both doctors and their patients into complacency, a feeling that the drug will do it all.

Recently we have re-discovered the benefits of non-pharmacological means of lowering blood pressure, means which often lead to a healthier lifestyle in general.

Rob Edwards' book is timely. It is based on his practical experience of working in a cardiac rehabilitation program and it is full of information which the lay person can understand and practical instructions which are easy to follow.

This is not a book by an over-enthusiastic zealot only interested in doing it his way. Rob Edwards has produced a balanced account of what can be achieved by relatively simple changes in diet, lifestyle and attitude.

Books like this will not result in our wholesale abandoning of drug therapy in hypertension; it may do even that in a proportion of patients, it may lead to smaller doses being used in others, but it should result in a healthier outcome for all.

Professor W. A. Littler, M.D., F.R.C.P.
Professor of Cardiovascular Medicine
University of Birmingham, United Kingdom

Introduction

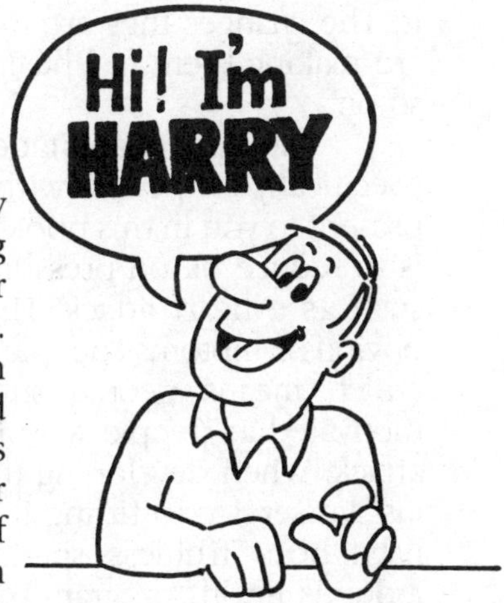

Gone are the days when the way people live is given only a passing glance of suspicion in the search for the cause of and cure for a disease. Lifestyle now takes the spotlight on centre stage in the prevention and treatment of many illnesses. This is particularly so for cardiovascular disease, the most common cause of disability and premature death in our community.

Almost one in every two Australians dies from heart disease or stroke. High blood pressure is one of the major causes. People with high blood pressure have up to four times the normal risk of developing heart disease and up to 15 times the normal risk of having a stroke. More than one million Australians have high blood pressure.

These very simple statistics are even more alarming if you consider that they could be greatly improved if people made relatively simple changes to their lifestyle. It's a tragedy to consider that the changes people need to make don't have to be a burden but rather they can make life more enjoyable. Yes, you can have fun lowering your blood pressure and avoiding its harmful effects — *you don't have to be a non-drinking, marathon running, vegetarian yoga instructor to enjoy the benefits of good health.* Sure, the changes you make need to be prudent enough to achieve health goals you set for yourself but they can also fit in with an enjoyable lifestyle. That's what this book is all about — taking action to improve your blood pressure and having fun at the same time.

My work in a cardiac rehabilitation centre has shown me both the devastation that high blood pressure can cause and also the vast improvement in the quality of people's lives when they take action to reduce their blood pressure. Even people who have had heart attacks tell me that they are getting far more out of life after their attack than they did before it. The changes they are making to avoid another heart attack are making them feel healthier, more active, less stressed and so on.

At the rehabilitation centre I developed a program specifically for people with high blood pressure which I now present to you in this book. The major objective of the program is to reduce blood pressure before it causes a serious illness, such as a heart attack. High blood pressure usually has no obvious symptoms (people may have it for years and not know) which means people suffering from it are often not as motivated as people who have had an illness such as a heart attack. When developing the program I had to pay more than just lip service to fitting it in with people's lifestyles. It would have been fruitless spending time developing yet another arduous health program that people rigidly stick to for a day, a week or even a year but slip back to the old ways when the 'health kick' is over. I set myself the challenge of developing a program that would be lasting, rather than producing yet another healthy dust gatherer for the book shelf. Part of the formula was to stop just telling people *what* they should do and devote more of my time to helping them work out *how* they might go about it. I spent much time reviewing and working through the difficulties people encountered in making lifestyle changes. I also had to be realistic and recognise the fact that most people (even authors of health books) enjoy not so healthy treats every now and then. In taking this approach it became clear to me that the real challenge was simple — to convince people that *good health and good fun go together.* I believe the rest will follow.

If someone were to ask you:

- would you like more enjoyment and happiness in your life?
- would you enjoy living your life with a minimum of suffering?
- do you want more vitality at work?

- would you enjoy extra healthy years in your retirement to watch your grandchildren grow up?

your answer would probably be an instinctive 'Yes'. If so, you really should believe that good health and good fun go together because these objectives are much more easily achieved if you are in good health.

This book is not simply for reading; all the reading in the world will not improve your blood pressure. It's what you *do* that counts. The book is designed for *doing*, yes, *doing* the things you can to position your problem of high blood pressure firmly into your past, rather than allowing it to remain a constant threat to your future health and happiness.

Better Blood Pressure is a 20 week (then lifelong) program of prudent yet realistic action to improve your blood pressure. The actions you will be taking are based on sound medical evidence which is promoted by physicians and preventive medicine associations worldwide. This book will be your work manual. It is written in a step-by-step fashion that leads you on a journey to achieving 'your aim'. You will be introduced to 'your aim' in chapter one.

Many people will gain impressive results from this program. Even so the program is definitely not a miracle cure that will ask you to disregard other forms of health care because it has arrived to save you. It's unfortunate that so many promise-filled miracle cures are offered these days. They can lead people to hop from one to another rather than identifying the lasting and sensible programs and sticking with them. Far too many miracle cures have failed at the expense and confusion of people who are genuinely trying to improve their health.

My experience has taught me not to tell people what I know but rather to provide them with information and tools that they can *use*. This book is a program of carefully designed and tested tools that you can *use* to improve your blood pressure. You will find the program is an enjoyable and genuine journey to greater quality of life and possibly more life itself.

I wish you well in reaping the rich harvest that good health has in store for you.

Robert J Edwards

Your Aim

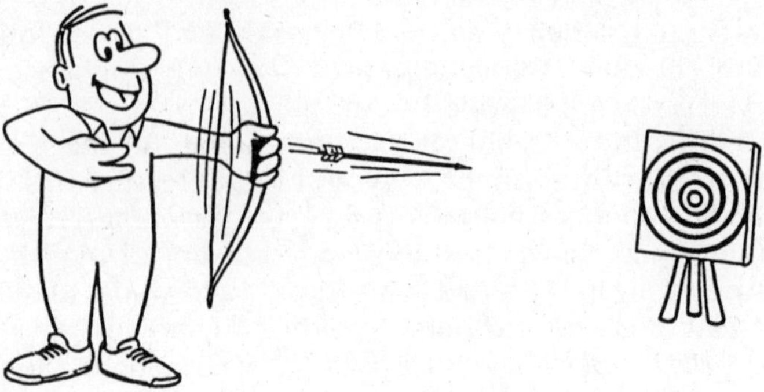

You are interested in this book probably because you:

- have high blood pressure;
- had high blood pressure which is now controlled by medication; or
- have normal blood pressure and want to keep it that way.

The ideal result of completing the program is to have normal blood pressure for the rest of your life without the need for blood pressure medication. Many will achieve this ideal result but it is unrealistic to expect it to be the automatic result of successfully completing the program. Before you begin, it is important that you have clear and realistic expectations of the results you hope to achieve. Whatever the situation 'your aim' is to:

reduce the risk high blood pressure is presenting to my future health and happiness

If you have high blood pressure you may expect it to reduce and if all goes to plan it will return to normal. If your blood pressure is normal because you are taking medication you may expect to reduce your need for medication and if all goes to plan you will have normal blood pressure without medication. If you are taking blood pressure medication but your blood pressure is still elevated you may expect it to return to normal without the need to increase your dose of medication. Then if all goes to plan you will be able to reduce and possibly eliminate your need for medication while maintaining normal blood pressure.

Most people who successfully complete the program will reduce their blood pressure to some degree. But, of course, things don't always go to plan and some won't achieve the ideal situation of lifelong normal blood pressure without the need for medication. You don't necessarily have to achieve this ideal situation to achieve your aim. If you adopt the guidelines in the program you will achieve your aim even if your blood pressure were to remain unchanged. 'How?' you ask.

The answer lies with the other risk factors that contribute to the development of diseases such as heart disease. High blood pressure is only one of several coronary risk factors. High blood cholesterol, smoking, being overweight, lack of exercise and stress are other risk factors that you have some control over. For example, by successfully completing the program it's likely that you will also lower your cholesterol level. If so you will have achieved your aim even if your blood pressure remains unchanged. The reason lies with the fact that risk factors don't work independently of each other. The effect of coronary risk factors is not simply added together: rather there is a multiplied effect. That means having high cholesterol, or any other risk factor, increases the health risk of having high blood pressure. Therefore if you lower your cholesterol, or improve other risk factors, you are genuinely lowering the risk that high blood pressure presents to your health.

The side effects of doing this program to improve your blood pressure are all good ones. They are so good the program may even be more important for those whose blood pressure improves only a little or not at all!

If you worry about yesterday's failures,
then today's successes will be few
ANON

You are the driver

Far too many people think they are leaving complete control of their blood pressure in the hands of their doctor. That's impossible. Doctors have a very important role to play in the management of high blood pressure, but they are not the ultimate controller — *you are.* You must accept responsibility for your health. It's solely your responsibility to manage it as you wish. That's fair because it's you who will live with the results of your management.

You are on a journey that you hope will lead you to enjoying or continuing to enjoy the benefits of good health. Consider doctors and other health professionals as sign posts beside the road on which you are driving. The sign posts give you information regarding the directions you should take, warnings about possible dangers and how far you have to travel — information to help *you* safely negotiate *your* journey. The sign posts are there to assist you but they do not do the driving for you. Whether or not you choose to use the information on the sign posts is entirely up to *you — you are the driver.* Whether or not you arrive safely at your destination is your responsibility.

This book is like a road map that you may use in conjunction with the sign posts.

Look forward to your destination
but don't forget to enjoy the journey
R.J.E.

Very Important!
This program is a valuable supplement to your normal medical care but it is not a complete replacement for it. Sure it's a good idea to aim to reduce your need for blood pressure medication but talk to your doctor about it first. Don't be tempted to toss your pills over your shoulder saying, 'I'll only do it the lifestyle way'.

Hypertension: What Does it Mean?

Understanding blood pressure and hypertension is really quite simple. The basic knowledge you will gain from this chapter will help you to work through the program in an informed fashion. The chapter is very brief so as to provide only the basic information you need to get on with the job. If you are interested in reading further about hypertension I encourage you to do so, but after you have allocated time to the much more important things *you can do* to improve your blood pressure.

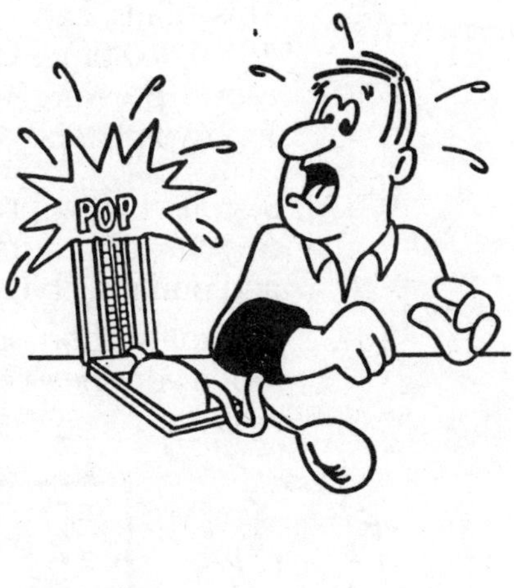

You know more than you think you do
DR. BENJAMIN SPOCK

What is blood pressure?

Blood is continually flowing around your body doing it's job delivering nutrients to, and removing waste products from your body's tissues. For this flow (circulation) to take place the blood has to be pushed. It must be put under pressure. The pressure that causes the blood to flow is called blood pressure. Blood pressure is generated by your body's pumping station, your heart. Your heart's very important job is to receive blood from the large veins and then to pump it out into the major arteries. Your heart may pump 10 000 litres of blood in a single day, enough to fill a small road tanker. To achieve an effective pumping action your heart continually goes through two phases:

- **The Systolic** (squeezing) phase is when your heart is contracting and pumping blood into the major arteries;
- **The Diastolic** (relaxing) phase is when your heart is relaxed and filling with blood. When it's full the next systolic phase begins and the cycle continues.

This filling and emptying process occurs as many as 1 000 000 times every week.
Blood pressure is generated by the heart so it also has two phases:

- Systolic blood pressure is the pressure of the blood in your major arteries when your heart is contracting and pumping blood into them;
- Diastolic blood pressure is the pressure in the arteries when your heart is relaxed and filling with blood.

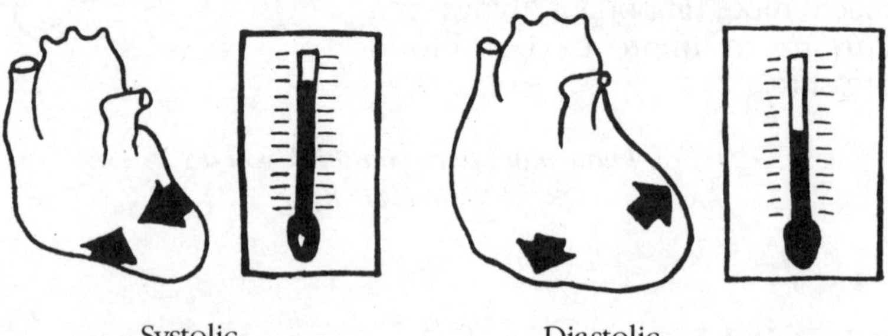

Systolic Diastolic

Try to find your pulse by holding your left hand out with palm facing upward, then place two fingers from the right hand on the upper and outer (thumb) side of your left wrist. You should be able to feel your pulse beating. Each beat is a surge of blood caused by a contraction of your heart. When you are feeling the actual beat, your blood pressure is in its *systolic* phase. The pause between pulses is when your heart is relaxed and filling with blood. This is when your blood pressure is in its *diastolic* phase.

When you have your blood pressure recorded it is expressed as two numbers which indicate the two phases of blood pressure. For example, your blood pressure might be 140/90 (expressed as 140 over 90). This means that your systolic blood pressure is 140 and your diastolic blood pressure is 90. Blood pressure is measured in the units — millimetres of mercury (mmHg). Throughout the program, blood pressure will be referred to simply by the numbers and the units will be assumed.

The only way to find out your blood pressure is to have it recorded.

What is normal blood pressure?

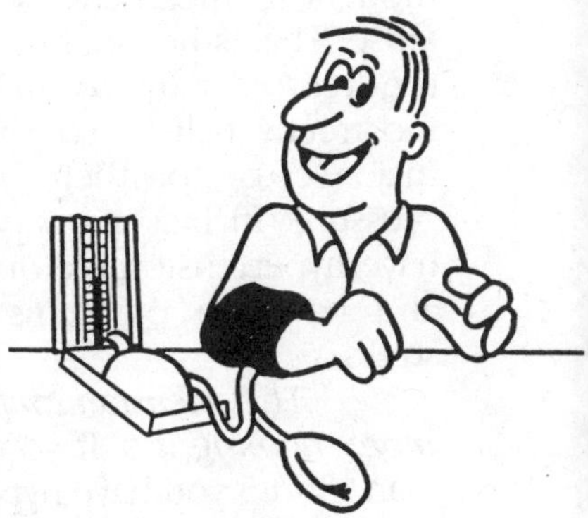

Most doctors consider systolic pressure of 140 or diastolic pressure of 90 to be the beginning of high blood pressure. In this program we will consider a systolic blood pressure from 100 to 135 to be normal and a diastolic blood pressure of 60 to 85 to be normal.

The risk of developing blood pressure related diseases reduces as blood pressure reduces. The lower your blood pressure is (without having symptoms of low blood pressure, called hypotension) the better. Reducing your blood pressure by any amount will be a worthwhile achievement.

Some people are concerned because their blood pressure fluctuates from one recording to the next. Don't worry, this is perfectly natural; your blood pressure is not meant to stay the same all day long. It is changing constantly in response to your body's changing needs. Just the same, it is important to be able to compare recordings so that you can be aware of any trends that may be occurring as you progress through the program. To collect meaningful records you will be averaging groups of recordings so as to even out the natural fluctuations. You should record your blood pressure under similar conditions. To do this, avoid vigorous exercise, smoking and alcohol for 30 minutes before each recording. Sit quietly for five minutes before taking the recording. Following these guidelines will allow you to confidently compare results over a period of time.

What is Hypertension?

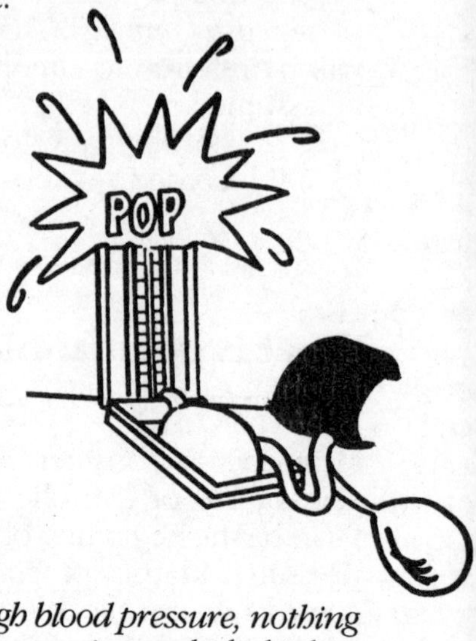

Hypertension is a word that frequently misleads people. It is often thought to mean stressed or being tense. This is not so, but is probably the reason why so many people incorrectly believe stress to be the major cause of their high blood pressure. In fact many people who have hypertension are quite relaxed and have no problems managing stress.

Hypertension simply means high blood pressure, nothing more, nothing less. If your blood pressure is regularly higher than 135/85 you have hypertension.

There are two types of hypertension:

- **Secondary** hypertension is due to a specific medical cause, for example kidney or hormonal disease. Approximately one in every ten people with high blood pressure has secondary hypertension. This program is not specifically aimed at people suffering from secondary hypertension. Just the same, if you have secondary hypertension and identify lifestyle factors that may adversely effect your health this program may be of value and possibly have a positive effect on your blood pressure. Indeed you may also achieve 'your aim'.

- **Essential** hypertension is probably the type of high blood pressure you have. It is not due to a specific medical cause but is most likely the result of lifestyle factors, or put more simply the way you live. This program is designed to address, in an enjoyable fashion, these lifestyle factors and in turn improve your blood pressure.

The life so short, the craft so long to learn
HIPPOCRATES

The Excessive 'S's: Be a Winner

Stacks of weight	**W**eigh less
Sittin' on ya bum	**I**ncrease activity
Schooners and scotch	**N**ot too much grog
Smokes	**N**ever
Salt	**E**ase back on salt
Stress	**R**elax

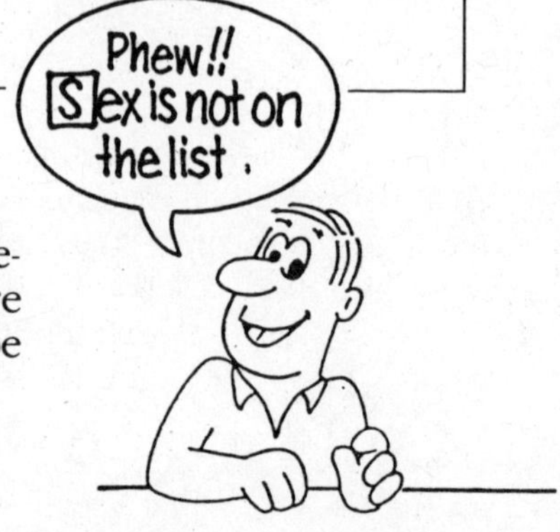

Hypertension may result from lifestyle factors. The Excessive 'S's are the six lifestyle factors that may be causing your high blood pressure.

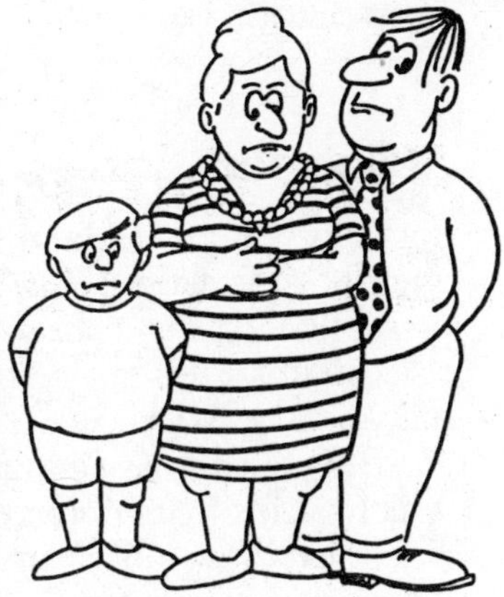

Stacks of weight

Excess body weight is a major cause of high blood pressure. Both systolic and diastolic blood pressure tend to go up as body weight increases. Even children who are overweight tend to have higher blood pressure than their leaner peers. Being overweight may also reduce the effectiveness of blood pressure lowering medication.

When people lose weight their blood pressure tends to decrease. Medical research tells us that weight loss is probably the most powerful non-drug tool available to address the enormous problem of hypertension in our community. In many cases, as people are losing weight, their blood pressure returns to normal before they reach their ideal weight. My personal experiences certainly support these claims.

Achieving normal weight has many other health benefits ranging from reducing the risk of developing diabetes and some cancers to making you better able to avoid run away buses.

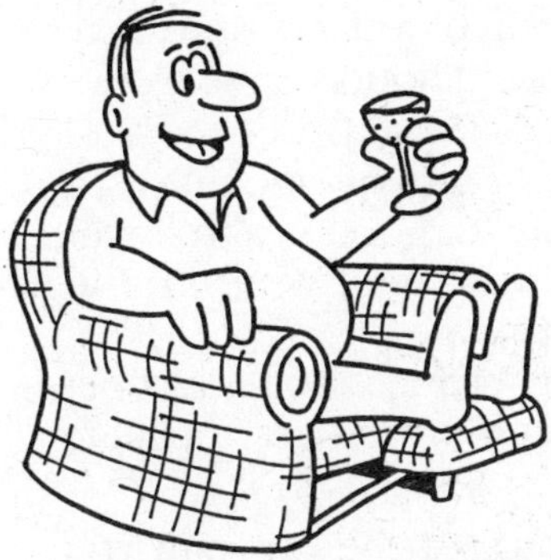

Sittin' on ya bum

If you don't take part in regular physical activity you probably are not as fit as you should be. Fitness has a direct effect on blood pressure; unfit people tend to have higher blood pressure than those who are fit.

Fitness also has indirect effects on blood pressure. Maintaining normal body weight is much easier if you are fit. Also regular exercise is one of the most powerful stress management tools you can employ. It's difficult to separate the direct and indirect effects of exercise but it doesn't really matter — sensible exercise is simply good medicine for blood pressure.

Schooners and Scotch

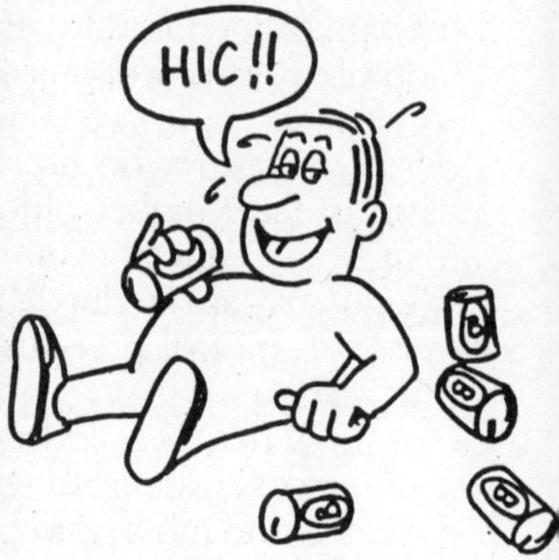

Some researchers claim that small amounts of alcohol may be cardio-protective, that is, it may reduce the risk of heart disease. This may or may not be so (keep your fingers crossed) but above a certain amount, which varies from person to person, alcohol clearly causes many serious illnesses. Among these illnesses is high blood pressure. Alcohol also has an indirect effect on blood pressure because it contributes to weight gain.

Many people who reduce the amount of alcohol they drink immediately reduce their blood pressure.

Smokes

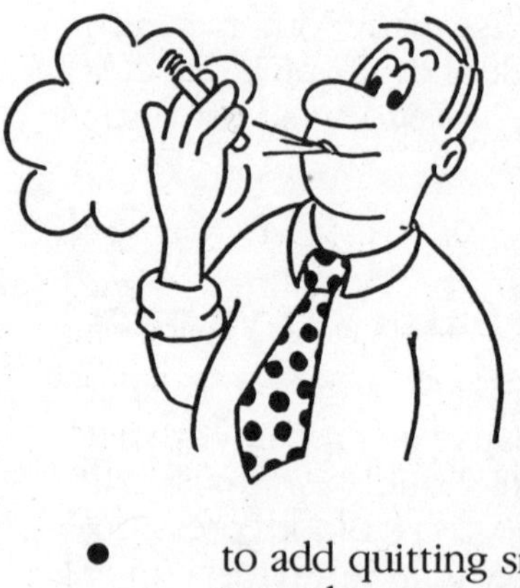

Smoking increases blood pressure at the time of having the cigarette and for up to 30 minutes after. This means if you smoke 20 cigarettes each day your blood pressure may be higher for ten hours than it would otherwise be.

Even though quitting smoking is a major priority for good health it will not be dealt with until Week 10. The reasons for this are:

- to add quitting smoking to the changes you are about to make may cause the program to be overwhelming and possibly not a success;
- when you are progressing through the program you will begin to feel more and more positive about yourself. You become better equipped to kick the habit because you will already be feeling healthier. Give yourself the time you need to prepare to quit forever.

From Week 1, record in Chart 5 'Quit Check List' the number of cigarettes you smoke each day.

Salt

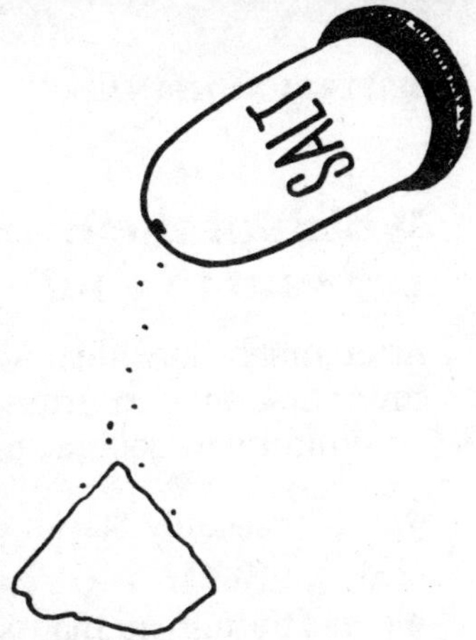

Salt is often thought to be the number one cause of high blood pressure. This is usually not the case. Certainly many people who reduce the amount of salt they eat do also reduce their blood pressure but, for most people, losing weight and getting fitter are more important.

Reducing the amount of salt you eat will not be addressed until Week 6 for two reasons:

- restricting salt may make the program unnecessarily difficult in the early stages;
- following the other Good Eating Guidelines, discussed later in the book, will inadvertently reduce the amount of salt you are eating.

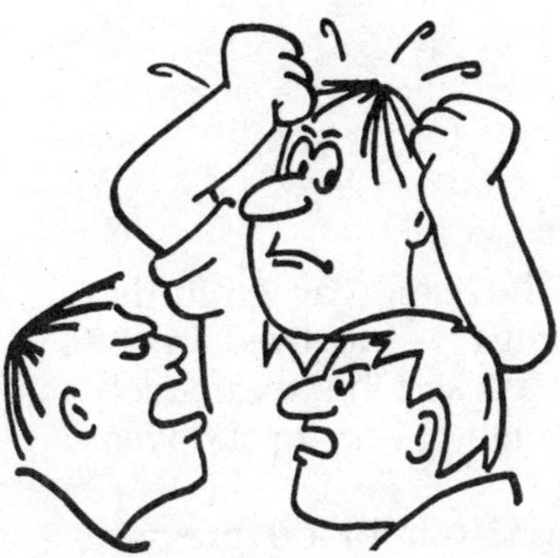

Stress

Some people hold stress solely responsible for their high blood pressure. This is rarely, if ever, the case. Stress does play a role in the development of high blood pressure but its indirect effects are probably more significant than the direct effects. People who are not coping well with stress are less likely to make health-conscious decisions in general, thus aggravating the other factors that contribute to the development of high blood pressure. Don't fall into the trap of blaming stress for your high blood pressure and neglecting other, probably more important, factors.

To find the cause is to begin the remedy
R.J.E.

Which of the Excessive 'S's is most relevant to you?

After much consideration of the available research and from my personal experiences I consider the order, for the community in general, to be as it is listed above:

- certainly Stacks of weight should be at the top of the list;
- though it may surprise some people Stress and Salt are rightly placed low on the list;
- Sittin' on ya bum rates highly on the list because of both its indirect and direct effects;
- the effect of Smoking on blood pressure places it in the middle of the list but it would be on top if we were considering health in general.

Of course, everyone is different and the order of importance of the Excessive 'S's may be quite different for you. When you have completed this chapter and your Self Assessment (see Record Section) you will have a feel for which of the Excessive 'S's are most relevant to you.

What about Family History!

Let's say Harry and I were born on the same day. From that day on we did exactly the same things — we lived in the same town, went to the same school, worked in the same job. We also ate the same healthy food, weighed 72.5 kg and were both physically fit.

Harry and I decided to record our blood pressure every day for one month. At the end of the month Harry's average blood pressure was 135/85 and mine was 115/70. The only difference between Harry and I is that we have different parents. Harry has inherited, from his parents, a tendency to have higher blood pressure than me. That's just how it is — you can't pick your parents.

One day Harry and I decide that this healthy lifestyle business is for the birds. For the next year we eat cream buns and meat pies with heaps of salt every day. We drink gallons of beer and good red wine and we do no exercise, not even a single walk around the block. At the end of the year we are both 98 kg and decide (after reading our own book) that we should check our blood pressures again. Harry's average result was 190/115 and mine was 140/90. Note the much greater leap in Harry's blood pressure. As well as inheriting a tendency to have higher blood pressure, Harry has also inherited a greater sensitivity to the lifestyle factors (the Excessive 'S's) that cause high blood pressure.

Some people can do all the right things and still have high blood pressure while others can do all the wrong things and have normal blood pressure. That's just how it is, but the critical point to remember is that if you have inherited the tendency to have high blood pressure you probably have also inherited a higher than average sensitivity to the Excessive 'S's. You need to be extra prudent to minimise the effect of these inherited traits.

I don't know who my grandfather was; I am much more concerned to know what his grandson will be
ABRAHAM LINCOLN

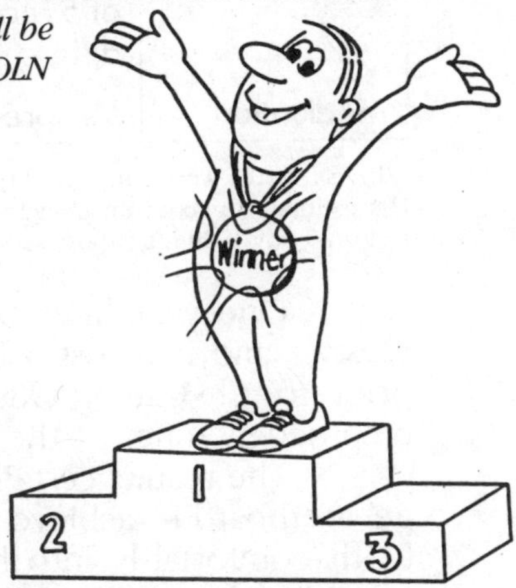

Be a winner

Being a winner is what this program is all about. Thousands of people have become winners. Lance is one such example. Lance is a 30-year-old supervisor working for a light industrial firm. Apart from having high blood pressure Lance was in good health.

Lance was concerned that he had high blood pressure at a relatively young age. He was particularly worried that his blood pressure was remaining elevated even though he was taking medication to control it. It appeared that Lance would have to take higher doses of medication. His doctor suggested he first consider the lifestyle factors that may be having an influence on his blood pressure — the Excessive 'S's. The doctor referred him along to our program. Lance took the advice and within four months he had eliminated his high blood pressure and was not using any medication. He quickly became a champion of lifestyle management of high blood pressure — he became a 'winner'.

LANCE'S PROGRESS		
	FEBRUARY 1989	JUNE 1989
Weight	93 kg	83 kg
Fitness	below average[1]	high
Alcohol	3–6 drinks per day.	Harry's Rule of Twos
Cigarettes	nil	nil
Salt	a little too much	moderately reduced
Stress	'managed OK'	more relaxed
Blood pressure	**149/104** (average of 5 recordings from different days)	**127/83** (average of 10 recordings from different days.)
Medication	Minipress 1 mg	nil

[1]Fitness scores were calculated from the results of exercise tests on a treadmill. His estimated maximum oxygen consumption was 41.5 mL/kg/min. At the re-test on 5 July 1989 his fitness score had risen to 54.0 mL/kg/min.

One year later Lance was maintaining his healthy lifestyle and had lost a further 2 kg. In the three months prior to Christmas 1989 Lance had his blood pressure recorded 37 times — the average recording was **128/74.**

The results certainly are impressive but Lance didn't go overboard to achieve them. The actions he adopted had to fit comfortably into his very busy lifestyle — a young marriage, demanding job and a part-time university course. He didn't have time for special 'health' meals that took hours to shop for and prepare, nor to spend two hours every day on an exercise bike (he went to the gym two to three times each week and some days walked or jogged to work), nor sit on a mountain and meditate every day.

Lance still has an occasional beer, he enjoys the exercise he does and he still goes out to dinner and treats himself. As well as fixing his blood pressure he is getting more out of life. He really did what you can do — make changes that fit your lifestyle in the long term.

The mould of man's fortune is in his own hands
BACON

What do you win?

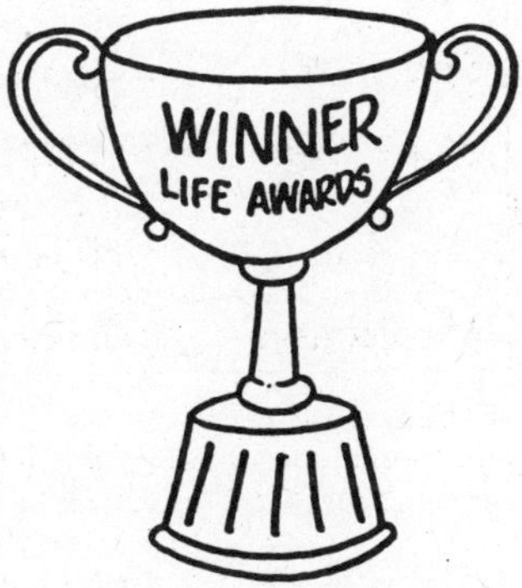

OK, if you become a winner, what do you win? What did Lance win? The prizes you win are greater than you may have ever imagined. Blood pressure is the major cause of stroke and one of the major causes of heart and kidney diseases. When you become a winner you reduce the risk of falling victim to these diseases. That means you stand to win two major prizes:

- **Quality of life!** If your life is free of these diseases you have a much greater capacity to enjoy it. That may mean being more effective at work or having more fun times with your grandchildren or pursuing your hobbies or travelling the world. Whatever it is that you enjoy doing, you will get more enjoyment out of it if you don't have to deal with the distresses of being unwell. Simply — you'll have more fun.
- **Life itself!** It might sound grand but it's true. Obviously, if you don't die prematurely as a result of these diseases you will live longer.

These prizes are of the highest quality but the effort required to achieve them is not at all unreasonable. Just for one minute shut your eyes and think about the effort and resources you devote to buying and maintaining your motor car or achieving goals at work or arranging a holiday. Think about the benefits you receive as a result of your efforts. Now think about the prizes you'll receive from becoming a winner. It is certainly worth the effort.

Health and love — the greatest investments listed on the stock market of life
R.J.E.

How it all works

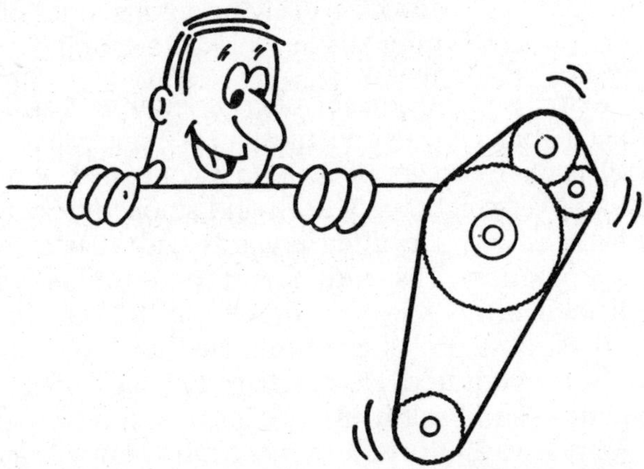

'Your aim' is now well established — *Reduce the risk high blood pressure is presenting to my future health and happiness.* It sounds great but you don't necessarily want to become a health fanatic to achieve it. You still want to enjoy life. After all what would be the point of being healthy but miserable? Switching to a healthier, and at the same time, more enjoyable lifestyle is easy if you are prepared to be:

- **Honest** with yourself — to fool another person is difficult but to fool yourself is a piece of cake (or was that two pieces).
- **Patient** — it has taken you years to develop high blood pressure. Accept that improving it is not an overnight job and that it may take several months to achieve worthwhile results. Quick cures are usually quick flops.
- **Flexible** — you will need to make some changes. Try to turn them in your favour and enjoy them. To 'grin and bear it' may not work in the long term.
- **Persistent** — it's a lifetime program so be careful not to get it all together only to let it slip away.

Add a small dose of commitment and this easy-to-follow step-by-step program will have you on your way to becoming a 'winner' and genuinely achieving your aim.

You're on the road to success when you realise
that failure is merely a detour
W.G. PLUNKETT

Some people devote much energy to learning about their health but neglect the most important aspect — what they can actually *do* about it. John is one such example. He was 30 kg overweight, very unfit and smoked heavily. He had a heart attack and shortly afterwards had a successful triple by-pass operation. His cardiologist and others who were assisting him in his recovery urged him to alter the lifestyle factors that most probably caused his heart condition. John became very motivated. He purchased many books on cardiac rehabilitation and healthy lifestyle and he studied them. When I met John I was surprised by how much knowledge he had acquired about his own health and how to improve it. I commented to him that he knew more about health than I did, but I was being paid to know it.

In 1989, eight years after John's first heart attack, he had his second. After his second attack he was unable to walk at a normal pace without getting serious heart pain (angina). He hoped for another by-pass operation but his heart was not in good enough condition for an operation to be successful.

Oh! by the way, when John had his second heart attack he was still 30 kg overweight, very unfit and smoked heavily. Yes, he learned and remembered plenty of healthy information and he enlisted the support of health professionals and he talked about and planned his health. But he didn't *do* it.

Though usually not as serious, this story is very common — people devoting energy in the wrong direction. Rather than identifying a few simple things they can *do* to improve their health and actually *doing* them. Again, this program is all about *doing* simple things to improve your health. It provides only the basic and necessary information you will need. You will have to look elsewhere to do an in depth study into the lifestyle management of high blood pressure. I encourage you to spend time expanding your knowledge about your health but after you have begun *doing* the things you can to improve your health.

Your Record Section

This book has a Record Section to help you actually *do* the program. The Record Section is your progress diary. You will make brief entries into the Record Section on a daily basis for the next 20 weeks. It only takes five minutes each day which is a valuable investment in your future.

Getting organised

If you are well organised the task of achieving your aim will be easy. As well as daily entries in your Record Section you will need to allocate time to complete each section of the program. To help you organise your program a Timetable (Chart 11) is provided in the Record Section. At the end of each chapter Harry will ask you to enter appointments into your timetable. If you follow Harry's directions and keep your timetable up-to-date you will have a smooth journey through the program.

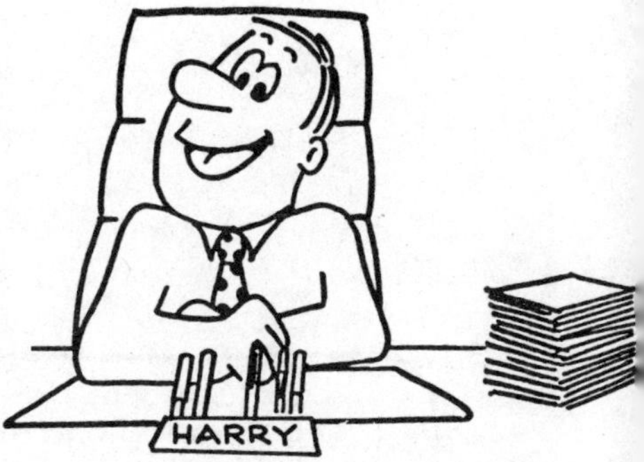

Some of the appointments you make will involve other people, for example your doctor. You are unlikely not to honour this appointment because you have committed his or her time. Involving a second person makes it relatively easy to honour appointments. On the other hand appointments that involve only yourself may be more easily missed. Ask yourself 'How often have I intended to do a job around the home but when the time came I let it slip by or put it off until another day?' The majority of appointments you make in the program will be with yourself. You will be simply allocating time to work through the various sections of the program. For some people these appointments, like the jobs around the home, may slip by or be put off until another day. It is most important that you don't allow this to happen. When you make a personal appointment, firmly commit yourself to it. Grant it the importance your health deserves and don't be distracted. When you make the appointment by writing it in your timetable also write it in your personal diary or on your wall calendar.

Make appointments for quiet times of the day when you are unlikely to be interrupted. You will make several appointments in the early stages of the program. Each will last between ten and 60 minutes.

If you are one of those people who is likely to let the appointments slip by, involve a second person. The ideal person would also have high blood pressure and be using the program as well. Alternatively family members or a friend may want to get involved to help you improve your blood pressure. The support of someone else may prove invaluable.

Organisation — the craftsman's tool in the trade of success
R.J.E.

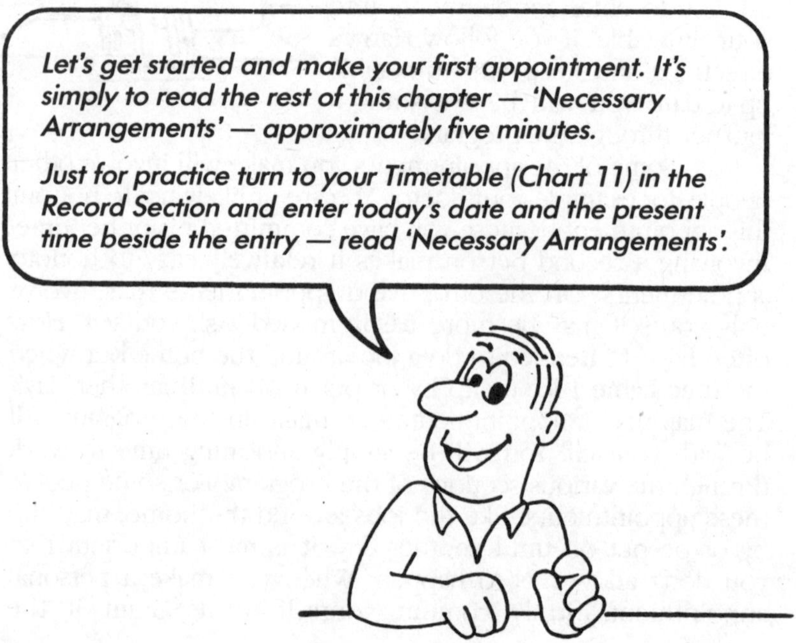
Let's get started and make your first appointment. It's simply to read the rest of this chapter — 'Necessary Arrangements' — approximately five minutes.
Just for practice turn to your Timetable (Chart 11) in the Record Section and enter today's date and the present time beside the entry — read 'Necessary Arrangements'.

Necessary arrangements

You will need to make arrangements to have your blood pressure recorded, weigh yourself and possibly see your doctor.

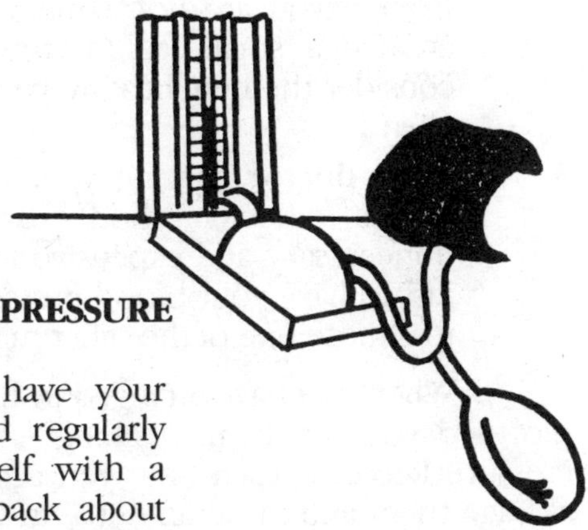

HAVING YOUR BLOOD PRESSURE RECORDED

If you can arrange to have your blood pressure recorded regularly you will provide yourself with a constant source of feedback about how you are progressing. This is not essential to the program but it does keep you tuned in and may help you stay motivated. There are several ways to have your blood pressure recorded regularly (two to six times per week):

- **Do it yourself.** This is the most convenient method to monitor blood pressure on a regular basis. Self monitoring blood pressure machines are available from many pharmacies. The machines are generally quite accurate and very simple to operate. The cost of reliable machines begins at about $100 which is not very expensive when you consider the convenience they provide. If you are in a private health fund you may be eligible for a rebate on the purchase price.

- **At work.** If your place of work employs a nurse ask him or her to record your blood pressure each day you are at work. As well as providing you with regular blood pressure recordings the nurse may become interested in your efforts to lower your blood pressure and offer valuable support. Don't be afraid to recruit supporters, their barracking may help you through some rough patches on the way to becoming a winner.
- **Gymnasiums and health clubs.** These usually have blood pressure recording facilities for their clientele. Even if you are not a member you may be able to arrange a small fee for the service. The staff may consider the new healthy you to be a prime potential client.
- **Your doctor.** Having your doctor involved in your efforts to lower blood pressure is valuable but it's unnecessary and expensive to see him or her weekly just to have your blood pressure recorded. It is better to choose one of the other methods.

When you have arranged to have your blood pressure recorded you can begin making entries in Chart 9 'Blood Pressure Records'. Each time you accumulate five recordings average them and make an entry in Chart 10 'Blood Pressure Graphs'.

You will never have any more time than you have today
W.G. PLUNKETT

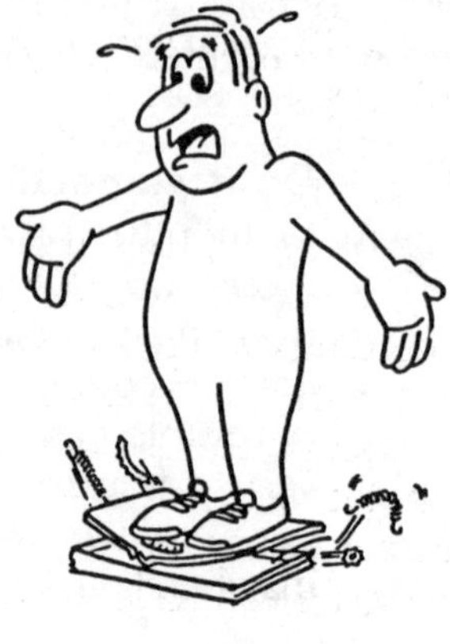

HAVING YOURSELF WEIGHED

Early in the program you will need to weigh yourself to establish if you are at your ideal weight or if you need to lose some weight. If you need to lose weight you will be weighing yourself about once every two weeks. Quality bathroom scales will be fine. Alternatively you may have access to scales at the same place as you are having your blood pressure recorded.

When you have arranged to have yourself weighed you can begin your two weekly entries in Chart 3 'Weight Loss Graph'.

INVOLVING YOUR DOCTOR

Your doctor may provide you with professional support and guidance as you progress through the program. An effective two-way relationship with your doctor is valuable. Involving your doctor is particularly important if you are over 35 and don't exercise regularly (you should see your doctor before taking up an exercise program — he or she may have important advice regarding the program). If you are taking medication for your blood pressure, it is particularly important that your doctor be involved.

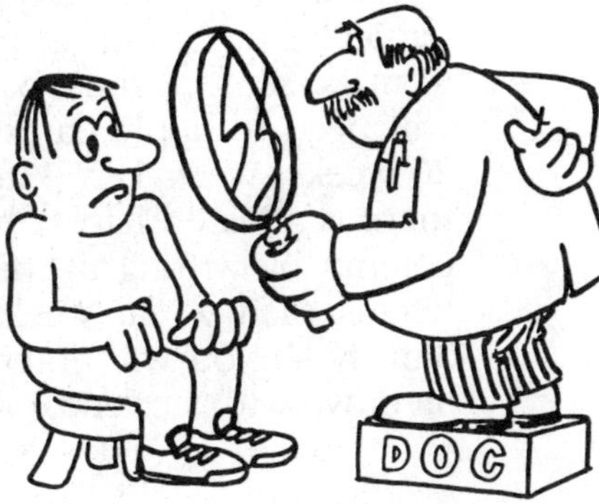

The program is based on a wealth of reliable medical research that has been conducted worldwide over the past 40 years. The principles you will be introduced to are supported by preventive medicine institutions around the world. The program is genuine so don't be afraid to seek your doctor's support. If you are unhappy with your doctor's response seek a second opinion.

Before seeing your doctor you will have, as much as possible, completed your Self Assessment. Your doctor may help you complete it by providing previous blood pressure recordings and discussing your medication with you.

Before making the appointment to see your doctor photocopy the 'Doctor's Information Sheet' below. Make the appointment in person so you can leave the sheet with the secretary. Ask the secretary to pass it on to the doctor so as he or she will have the opportunity to read it before you arrive for the actual appointment. The Doctors Information Sheet informs your doctor that you are doing the program and provides a brief summary.

A little support — a big difference
R.J.E.

PREPARING YOUR RECORD SECTION

The Record Section requires you to make simple entries at particular times during the program. For the Record Section to make sense it must be given a relevant time frame — you will need to apply dates to it. The program is divided into 20 weeks, Week 1, 2, 3 and so on. Alongside your Timetable there is a Date Chart (Chart 12). You will complete the right column by writing in the date of the particular Sunday that begins each week. Week 1 of the program will begin next Sunday so you will enter next Sunday's date beside Week 1. Sit down with a calendar and write all the dates in.

SELF-ASSESSMENT

The Self Assessment is a comprehensive review of your health in terms of the factors that may be contributing to your high blood pressure. You will do a Self Assessment at the beginning of the program and after Week 20 (and as often as you like in the future). The *before* Self Assessment will assist you in identifying what factors may be contributing to your high blood pressure. The *after* Self Assessment will indicate how well you have progressed.

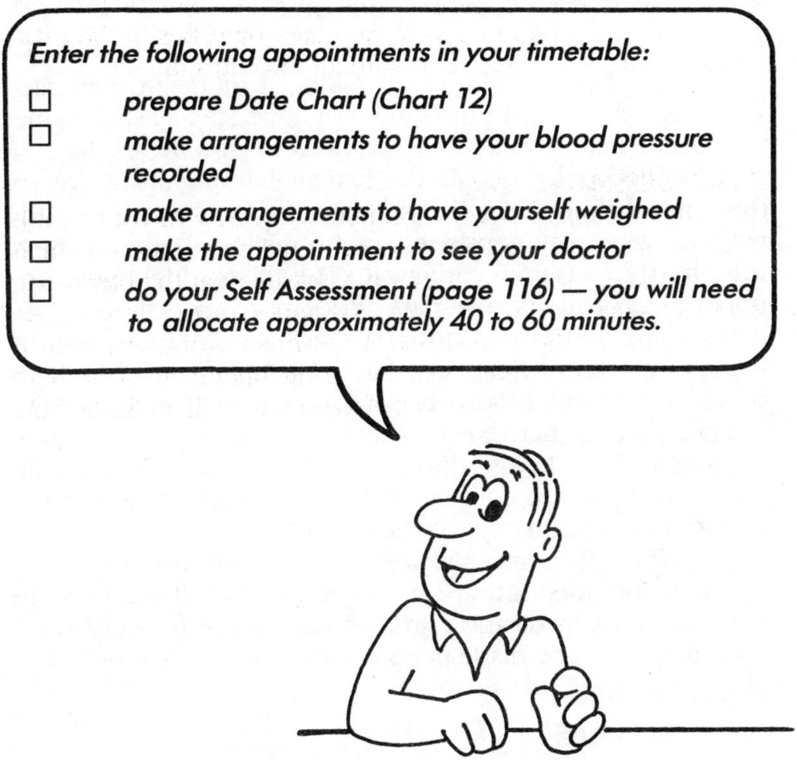
Enter the following appointments in your timetable:
☐ prepare Date Chart (Chart 12)
☐ make arrangements to have your blood pressure recorded
☐ make arrangements to have yourself weighed
☐ make the appointment to see your doctor
☐ do your Self Assessment (page 116) — you will need to allocate approximately 40 to 60 minutes.

Doctor's Information Sheet

The patient presenting this sheet is taking part in a self-help program to improve blood pressure. The program is conducted by way of the patient working through the publication *Better Blood Pressure*, written by Robert Edwards and published by Sally Milner Publishing. The program is based on widely accepted research evidence. It is designed as a supplement to traditional medical care, not a replacement for it.

The objectives of the program are:

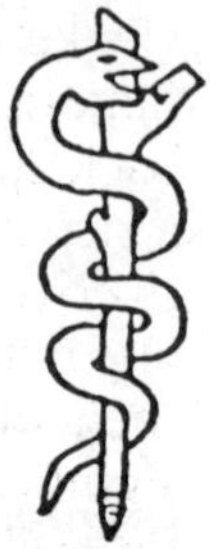

- achievement and maintenance of ideal weight
- improved physical fitness
- moderation of alcohol consumption
- smoking cessation
- moderation of salt consumption
- improved stress management

Emphasis is placed on taking a moderate approach which is sustainable in the long term. The step-by-step format will enable many to achieve these healthy objectives.

The book suggests the patient inform you by way of this information sheet, that he or she is taking part in the program. You may consider it worthwhile to take an active role in the patient's program. The book highlights the importance of an effective patient-doctor relationship.

The patient conducts a Self Assessment at the beginning and conclusion of the program. You may assist by providing previous blood pressure records and comments. The lifestyle changes may have some positive side effects such as improved blood lipids, glucose and uric acid. If these results are available or you consider them to be worthwhile pursuits could you provide a copy to the patient.

The program supports a goal of reduced anti-hypertension medication. At the same time it stresses the importance of medication and strongly suggests decisions to alter medication be made in consultation with a doctor.

In good health,

Robert J Edwards

Weigh Less

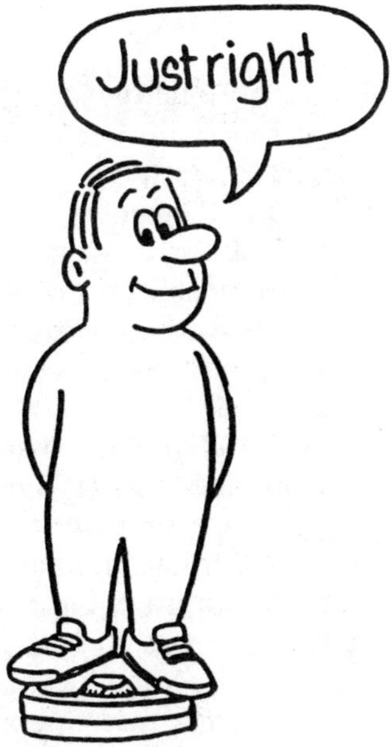

It was recognised as early as the 1940s that losing weight improved blood pressure. Dr Walter Kempner (Duke University Medical Centre) is famous for his research on the topic back in those early years. He used a rice and fruit only diet to get very overweight patients to lose weight. He noted that as they lost weight their blood pressure often reduced significantly. He also noted that many with heart and kidney disease improved their conditions as well. This was the first of many studies that proved beyond any doubt that there is a strong link between being overweight and having high blood pressure. Modern research has shown that weight loss as small as 3 kg can noticeably reduce blood pressure. You will be comforted to know that modern research has also shown that a prudent diet can be much more enjoyable than just rice and fruit.

The reason why being overweight causes high blood pressure is unclear but it is most probably related to the fact that blood volume increases with body weight. Extra fat tissue needs to be supplied with blood. It is estimated that one extra kilogram of fat requires an extra 2000 metres of blood vessels. That simply means more work for the heart and possibly high blood pressure is a result.

Losing weight and keeping it off

If you have chosen to lose weight, it is essential that you choose a method that is lasting. Fiona is just one of many people who chose quick cure methods with disappointing results.

Fiona decided she needed to lose about 30 kg. In the year following her decision she lost 50 kg. The problem was that in the same year she also gained 53 kg. She lost 16, gained 17, lost 21, gained 23, lost 13 and finally gained 13 kg. The result of her enormous efforts was a net weight gain of 3 kg. The monetary cost of her efforts was $3000. The personal cost was also great because by the end of the year Fiona's self-esteem and belief in her ability to have a normal weight was shattered.

What went wrong? It's not as though she was not trying. She was trying in the wrong direction. She chose a quick cure method that had no hope of ever being a part of her normal lifestyle. The quick cure programs always have an end point where you go back to normal. The key to successful weight loss is starting with only moderate changes that will become 'normal'.

How many people do you know who have lost weight only to put it back on? How many times have you heard people say 'I've only one week (or two kilos) to go on my diet and I can start eating normally again' or 'I am going to go on a diet for a while and lose this extra weight'? For a weight loss program to be successful it must be a manner of eating and level of exercise that is similar to what you intend doing for the rest of your life. Certainly some changes are necessary but the changes must be reasonable.

Sure, when you change old habits there are some bumpy patches but for long-term success the changes must be able to settle down to a situation that will be lasting. If someone asked you in one year from now 'Are you on a diet?', your answer needs to be 'No, not really — I did make some changes to my eating habits some time back but it's now simply what I do.' This is what the Good Eating Guidelines are all about.

- **Forget** the high flying expensive programs with the fat *before* and skinny *after* pictures in the window.
- **Forget** the quick cure diets
- **Forget** counting every single calorie you eat
- **Forget** all your past efforts.

You are starting anew. Your Healthy Eater's Creed will help you on your way:

HEALTHY EATER'S CREED
My past efforts to lose weight are past, I am making a fresh start.
I will lose weight by sticking to the 'Good Eating Guidelines' and 'Increasing Activity'.
I will be patient because I know slow, steady and forever is best.
I am realistic and expect to have some bumpy patches as I change my old habits but I will persevere until I succeed.
I will have the occasional treat and enjoy it without feeling guilty.
I genuinely believe in myself and my ability to lose weight and keep it off.
So what, if I slip up and put a couple of kilograms back on! I'll just keep working at it because these slip-ups are not major failures, just minor detours on my road to success.
I am going to enjoy the new healthy me.

Now, show yourself that you are serious by reading it out loud.

Weight loss — the basics

Weight loss is achieved by altering your energy balance. Food energy is measured in kilojoules (calories in old money). You take in food energy when you eat. Your body uses up food energy to function.

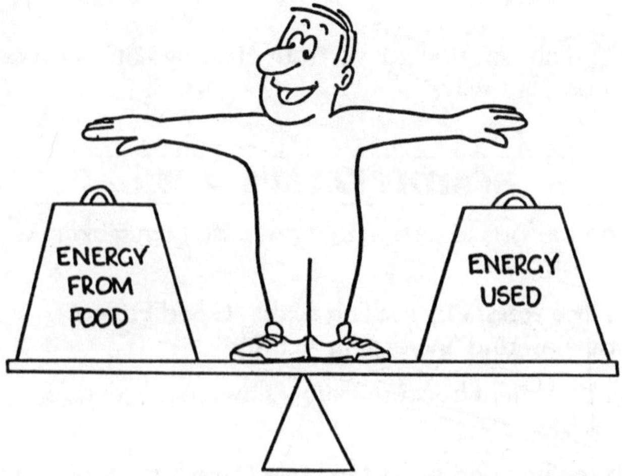

When the amount of energy your body takes from the food you eat is the *same* as the amount of energy your body uses to keep itself functioning, you remain the *same weight.*

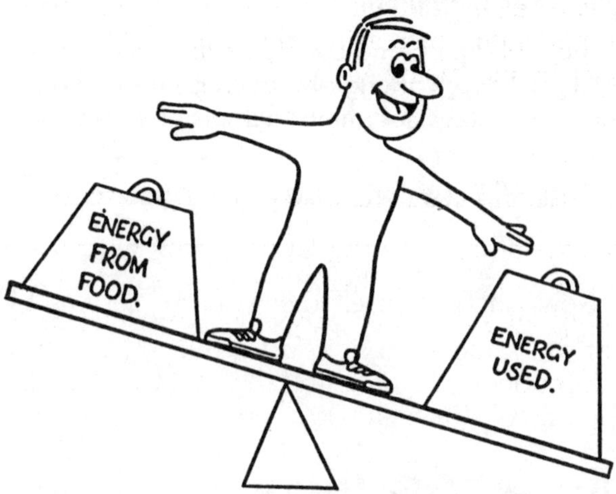

When the amount of energy your body takes from the food you eat is *less* than the amount your body uses, you will *lose weight.* The extra energy your body needs is taken from your stores of body fat.

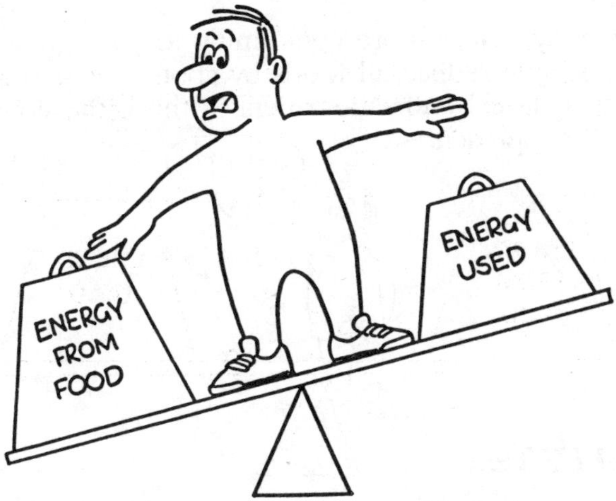

When the amount of energy your body takes from the food you eat is *more* than the amount your body uses, you will *gain weight*. The leftover energy is stored as body fat.

You will be moderately reducing the amount of food energy you eat by following the Good Eating Guidelines. You will be moderately increasing the amount of food energy your body uses by Increasing Activity.

But what if I am already at my ideal weight?

You should still stick to the Good Eating Guidelines because they are the basis for healthy eating for everyone in the community. If you are at your ideal weight you simply eat more of the same food, if you feel like it. You may need to be extra prudent in addressing the other factors that may be contributing to your high blood pressure.

What if I stick to the guidelines and don't lose weight?

This would be surprising, particularly if you also increased your activity level. If in six weeks your weight has not changed, check closely that you are conforming to your guidelines. If you are, simply reduce all foods by about 10% and increase your activity level by 10%. Be patient — this is the slow, steady and forever approach.

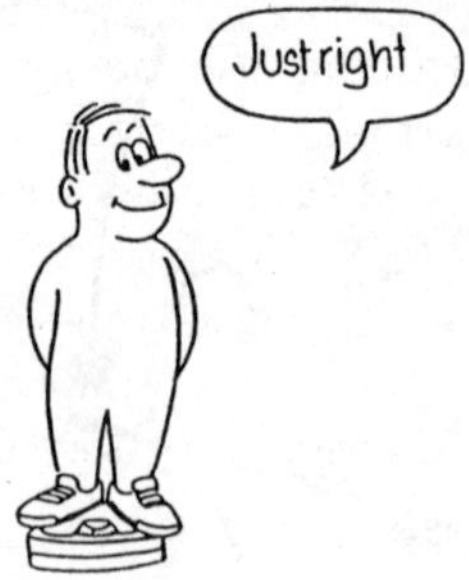

The SELF Test

It is most important that before you make any lifestyle changes you give careful consideration to the way you are going to approach the situation. Before making a particular change, whether it be dietary or otherwise, give it the SELF Test. The SELF Test removes some of the inflexibility and harshness that often accompanies lifestlye change, in particular changes to your eating habits.

The actions you take have to be prudent but they must also be:

- as **Simple** as possible.
- as **Easy** as you can make them.
- **Lasting Forever,** which means the actions must fit comfortably into your daily activities.

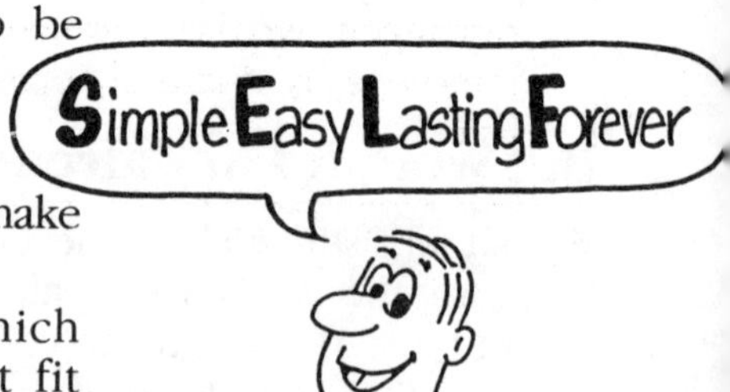

So whatever changes you make give them the **SELF** Test.

Harry and I really enjoy barbecued sausages but we are aware that they are very fatty and contain the particular type of fat that may increase our cholesterol. For an example let's give sausages the **SELF** Test:

SIMPLE — We don't eat sausages, we don't buy them and we don't cook them. That's simple and clear.

EASY — We still go to the butcher's shop but rather than ordering sausages we choose a leaner cut of meat. The meal that is cooked has less fat than sausages, but has lost very little in its appeal. We made the change as easy as possible. To go on a 'health kick' and decide meat is out altogether and replace the sausages with bean sprouts would make the change difficult.

LASTING FOREVER — Harry and I have been invited to a friend's place for a barbecue. We arrive and detect the delightful smell of barbecued sausages and soon find that they are the only meat available. What do we do? We have a couple and enjoy them as a treat. We don't feel guilty because we know that guilt is one of the greatest enemies against us leading a reasonably healthy lifestyle. We certainly don't arrive waving a lettuce leaf in one hand and a carrot stick in the other proclaiming we are on a special blood pressure diet. Doing this would make us feel uncomfortable and there is a good chance we would dump the diet there and then. Certainly if the barbecue was a regular event we would have to intervene by discretely providing our own lean meat or fish.

Good Eating Guidelines

Your Good Eating Guidelines are divided into five sections: Eating more fibre; Eating less fat; Low fat cooking; Eating less sugar; Ease back on salt (separate chapter).

Work through each section and highlight or circle the guidelines that you are not already conforming to (a highlighter pen is useful). When you have identified all the guidelines that are relevant to you turn to your Record Section and highlight the Good Eating Guidelines Check List (Chart 2).

Eating more fibre

Dietary fibre is currently experiencing an upsurge in popularity. The reason is largely because of a specific type of dietary fibre that may have a positive effect on blood cholesterol. This may be good news for some people with high cholesterol but please don't forget fibre's most important role is to keep you regular. We don't often talk about it, but eating plenty of fibre insures that you are regularly (preferably daily) producing large, soft stools. This significantly reduces your risk of developing several diseases including the following:

- **Haemorrhoids** are much more common than most people realise. One of the major reasons why haemorrhoids develop is the extra effort required to eliminate dry and slow moving stools.
- **Diverticulitis** may be caused by large dry stools distorting the wall of the bowel. The illness can be quite serious but could be, in many cases, avoided by eating a high fibre diet.

- **Bowel cancer** may be caused by slow moving stools keeping cancer-causing agents in contact with the bowel wall for longer than they otherwise would. Eating more fibre can markedly reduce your chance of developing this killer disease.

Some types of dietary fibre such as oat bran, baked beans, lentils and so on *may* help reduce blood cholesterol. If your cholesterol is elevated, including these foods may be useful but losing weight and improving fitness are usually much more important.

Dietary fibre also plays an indirect role in the blood pressure story. Fibre is filling without being fattening so if you eat high fibre foods instead of fatty foods you will find it easier to lose weight.

EATING MORE FIBRE GUIDELINES

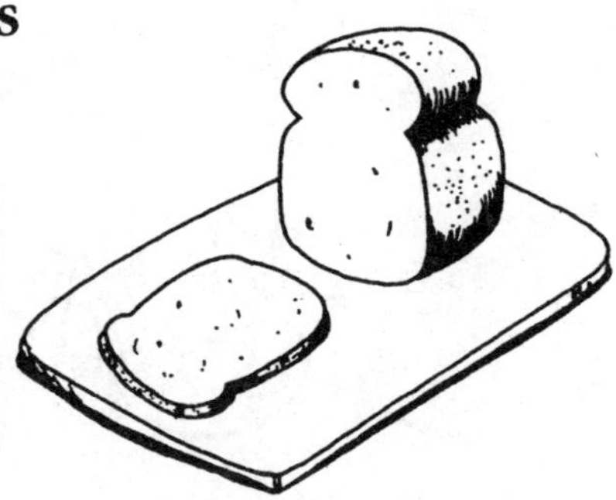

1. DO use wholemeal or wholegrain bread. If you don't eat wholemeal or wholegrain bread highlight this guideline. Males: four to eight slices per day; females: two to six slices per day. Bread rolls are equal to two slices of bread. Two cracker breads may substitute for one slice of bread.

Wholemeal is best as it contains most fibre. Wholegrain ranks second. White bread is not an unhealthy food but it has very little fibre thus does not provide the benefit of adding fibre to your diet.

In the past, bread has had a bad image as a fattening food. This is not the case. It's what we put on it that gives it the bad name. If you decide to eat more because you are hungry, bread is a good choice. Remember you don't need to be hungry to lose weight.

I am reluctant to limit the quantity of bread you consume because it is a good filling food. Usually the 'Eating Less Fat' guidelines and 'Increasing Activity' are sufficient to get your weight steadily reducing. Remember you don't need to be hungry — fill up on fruit, veges and bread.

2. DO include a variety of fruits.
Two to six pieces every day. If you eat less than two pieces of fruit highlight this guideline.

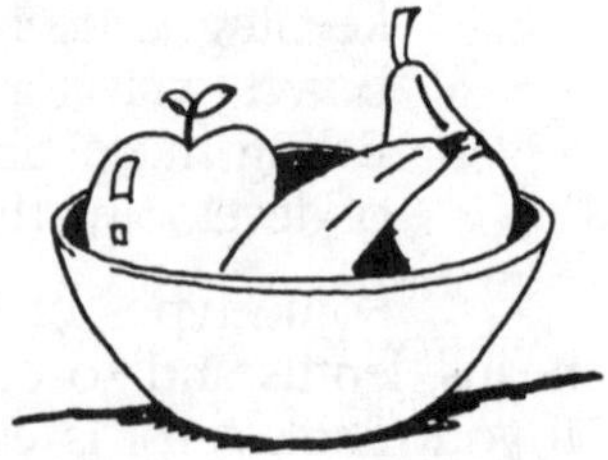

Fruit is a great substitute for the high energy foods that may be causing you to be overweight. Reach for a mango instead of a chocolate bar, strawberries instead of lollies, fruit salad instead of ice-cream for dessert.

If you have not been a regular fruit eater be careful not to fall into the trap of buying just apples and oranges and becoming bored. Be adventurous and try plums, fresh pineapple, kiwi fruit, mangos, grapes and bananas, for example.

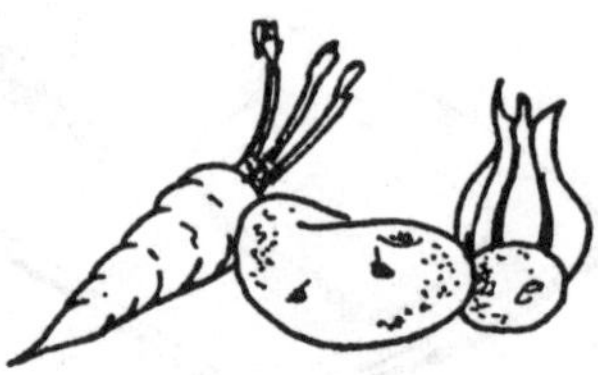

3. DO eat plenty of vegetables.
At least three servings each day. If you are eating plenty of fruit and vegetables you are probably eating less fat. Choose a variety of vegetables, including salad vegetables. Avoid oil when cooking vegetables and keep cooking time to a minimum. Try some vegetables with their skin on for extra fibre.

If you buy canned or frozen vegetables avoid those prepared with fats, oils or salt. That means oven fry chips are out.

4. DO eat a high fibre breakfast.
A high fibre breakfast fills you up and helps you avoid snacking on fattening foods before lunch. Try cereals, wholemeal toast or fruit for interesting and very filling breakfasts. See Harry's Healthy Hints (page 86) for some ideas.

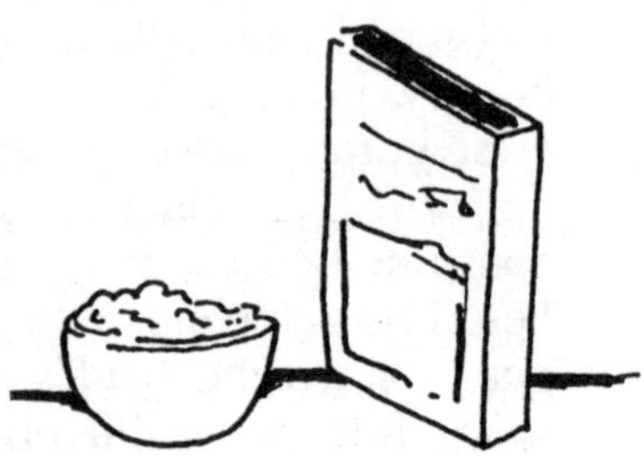

5. DO use pasta and rice. Wholemeal pasta and brown rice are the best choices because they contain plenty of fibre. Try them but if you don't enjoy the wholemeal varieties continue to use white pasta and white rice. White varieties are still valuable in a healthy diet because they are low in fat and are very filling.

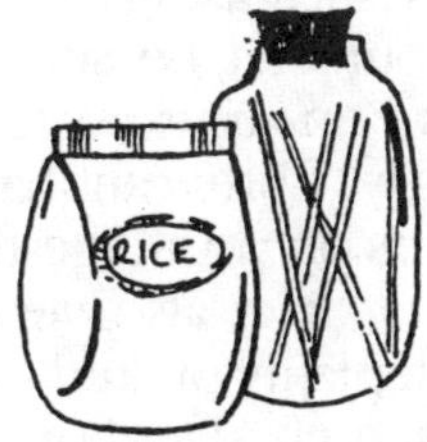

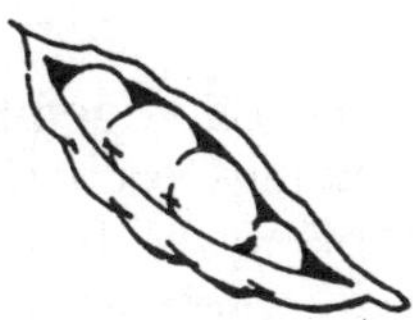

6. DO try some dishes with beans or lentils. Beans and lentils are packed with fibre, some of which may be helpful in lowering cholesterol. Include them in your day to day eating. It's as simple as serving baked beans, bean salads, plain old green peas; toss a handful of lentils into a stew or casserole. You may also consider making meals that are based on beans, such as Minestrone or Veal and Chick Pea Casserole. See the recipe section.

7. DO eat fruit and vegetables in preference to their juice. Limit juice to one glass per day. The problem with juice is that it is easy to drink because all the fibre has been removed. You take in a lot of food energy for very little satisfaction. For example six large apples have the same amount of energy as two glasses of apple juice — try eating six apples in 30 seconds.

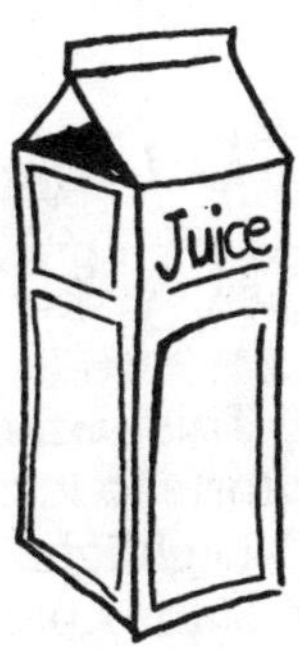

When increasing the amount of fibre in your diet be sure to do it gradually. An unexpected increase in dietary fibre can have spectacular effects on your digestive system.

It is also very important to drink plenty of fluid — eight or more cups each day. Have a drink with each meal — it helps fill you up.

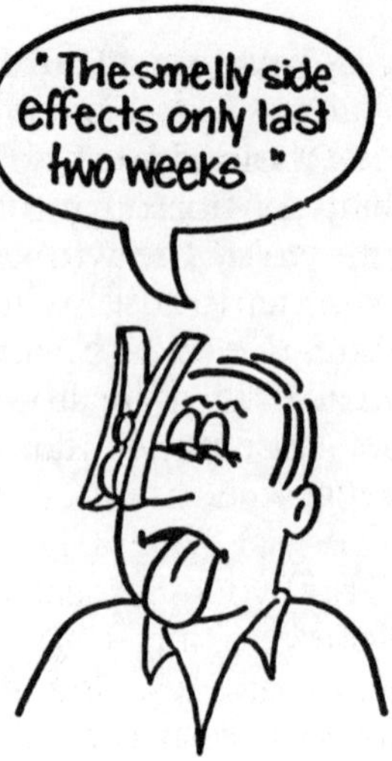
"The smelly side effects only last two weeks"

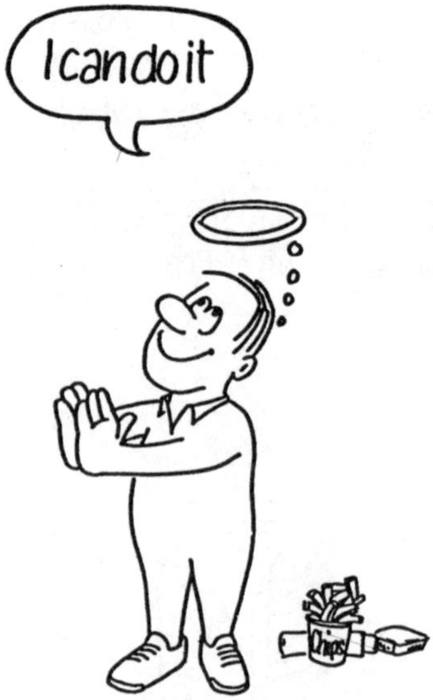
I can do it
Chips

Eating Less Fat

Some fat in your diet is important but only small amounts are required to meet your body's needs. Fats and oils have the highest amount of energy per gram of any food, which is why they are the major reason people put on unwanted weight. Ten apples, four wholemeal salad rolls and a 3 kg pumpkin have the same amount of energy as four sausages, a meat pie and 90 ml of olive oil. Fat makes you fat because you can eat lots of it easily.

This section will probably be the most important in your efforts to lose weight.

Highlight, in your Good Eating Guidelines Check List (Chart 2) the guidelines that you don't already conform to.

EATING LESS FAT GUIDELINES

8. DO buy low fat ingredients. When you are buying food be very selective and try to always return home with a low fat shopping basket. Choose, for example, best mince rather than sausage mince or lean steak rather than fatty chops. You may choose a cut such as pork chops that have a large amount of fat but you can easily remove it before cooking. Choose low fat yoghurt instead of the full cream varieties, and natural muesli rather than toasted, as toasted muesli often has added oil. Choose tuna canned in brine rather than oil. (Preferably salt reduced brands and drain well before using.)

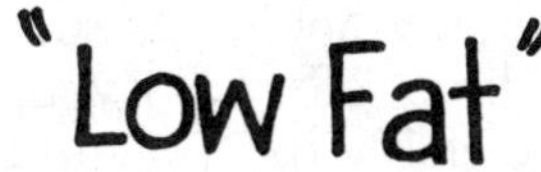

Take a little extra time to shop and always ask yourself 'Is there a low fat alternative?'

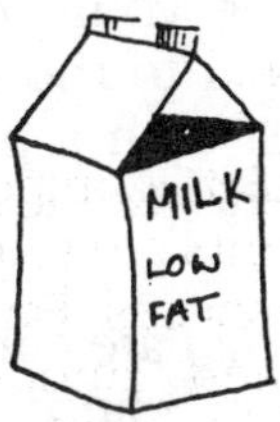

9. DO use skim or low fat milk. Skim and low fat milks are best because they contain almost no fat. There are also a variety of reduced fat milks available. They have considerably less fat than whole milk and are a good stepping stone to using the low fat varieties.

10. LIMIT the amount of all oils you use. Where possible avoid using oil or fat when preparing food. If you do need oil use it as sparingly as possible. If you buy more than 500 ml of cooking oil for a family of four every two months you are using too much.

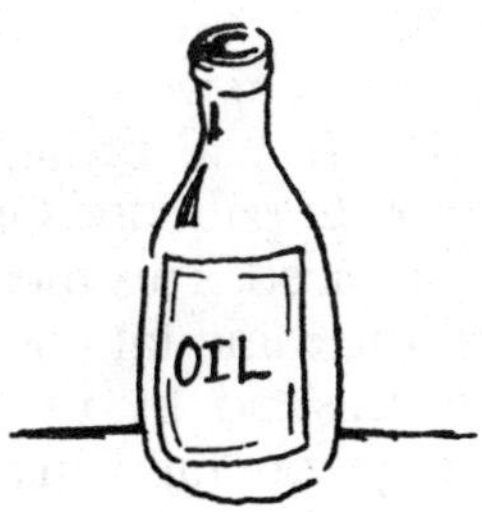

People are often confused by the advertising of some oils. The adverts leave you believing that it is a good thing to eat copious amounts of the particular brand. This is not so, all oils and fats have the same amount of energy per gram which means that olive oil or dripping will have the same effect on weight gain. Certainly fats such as lard, dripping and copha may have a direct effect on your cholesterol so they are best avoided. Preferably use polyunsaturated or mono-unsaturated oils but don't be mislead by the advertising that tells you they are good for you. Losing weight and increasing activity are far more powerful tools for reducing cholesterol than any oil on the market.

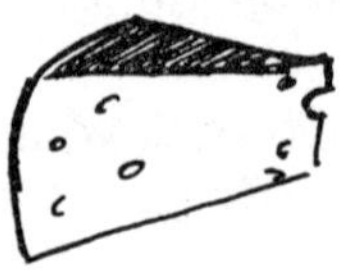

11. LIMIT cheese. If you are a cheese lover you will need to put it in its correct place — as a treat. Avoid cheese on biscuits or on sandwiches or slicing that chunk off the block as you walk past the fridge. Be sure to have something else at hand to nibble on. It's a dangerous time for your weight when habit takes you to the fridge in search of that cheese snack. Treat yourself with a punnet of strawberries, a pear, a mango or whatever healthier alternative suits you.

What about the 'reduced fat' cheeses that are currently making advertising agents wealthy. These cheeses are portrayed to be a cheese lover's godsend. You can be easily tricked. A cardiac patient, Paul, with whom I was working had chosen to eat only two slices of cheese per week. One day he happily exclaimed to me that he had found a cheese that he really enjoyed and it was also healthy (that's what the advert said). He had brought the packaging in for me to show to the other patients. On close examination the cheese was 30% fat reduced. This meant three slices of the reduced fat cheese had the same fat content as two slices of normal cheese. Paul was mislead by the glossy advertising and was innocently eating more fat than previously when he was eating the normal cheese. Sure you can eat a little more of the reduced fat varieties — but only a little more.

Low fat and reduced fat cheeses:

- Less than 5 g of fat per 100 g of cheese is *fine.*
- 5 to 10 g of fat per 100 g of cheese use *in moderation.*
- 10 to 15 g of fat per 100 g of cheese *be very sparing.*
- 15 g or more is a *special treat.*

Most cheeses have the fat content on the packaging. If buying cheese off the block ask the person behind the counter.

Cheeses that are less than 5 g of fat per 100 g should be your preference. They are cottage, low fat ricotta and some low fat hard cheeses made of skim milk. Some people enjoy these cheeses while others don't. Try them several times before putting them on the 'no way' list but don't persevere with something you truly dislike. You may find these cheeses useful in cooking.

Advertising may be described as the science of arresting human intelligence long enough to get money from it
STEPHEN LEACOCK

12. LIMIT butter and margarine.
Spread very thinly. Use the 'tuck-shop spread' — that is, spread it on then scrape it off. If the filling for your sandwich or toast is moist you don't need any butter or margarine at all.

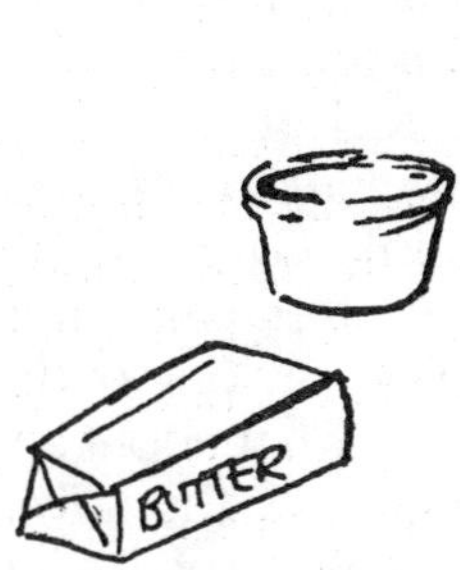

Butter or margarine — which is best? They both contain the same amount of energy per gram but margarine is preferred because of the type of fat it is, and it is usually easier to spread thinly.

This guideline may seem unimportant but if you look more closely it may rank as one of the most important. If you currently use 500 g of margarine every two weeks and decided to cut in half the amount you eat, you would eat 6.5 kg less fat each year as a result. That's 65 kg less fat over the next ten years. It really does add up. Reduced fat margarine is a healthier choice but you must still be sparing.

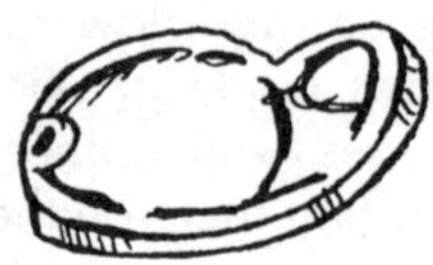

13. AVOID fatty meats. Choose lean cuts of meat or cuts that you can easily remove the fat from before cooking. Avoid sausages, fatty chops, bacon, salami, devon and most pressed meats. This is a very important guideline and may have a major impact on your weight.

14. AVOID cream, sour cream and ice cream. These are very high in fat and are best avoided.

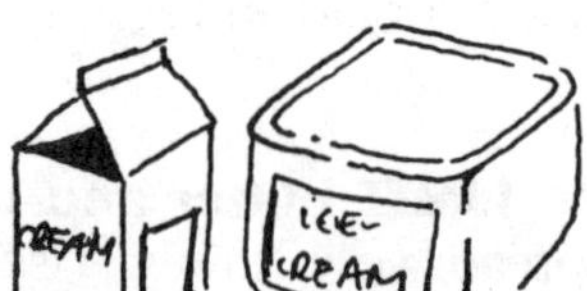

Be particularly careful of ice cream as it also contains a large amount of sugar — have two scoops per week as a real treat. You may prefer an ice cream on an outing but certainly avoid that serve of ice cream after each meal. If you are a regular ice cream eater it's probably one of the main reasons why you are overweight.

What about all the new supposedly healthy ice creams? Like cheese, the advertising can lead you astray. For example low cholesterol ice cream doesn't necessarily mean that it's low fat or that it's not loaded with sugar. Be wary when you shop. It's best to have the real thing for the odd treat and truly enjoy it.

15. AVOID eating biscuits, cakes and pastries. Such delightful traps that so often keep those extra kilos where they are. Put them back into their rightful place — as a treat. Cakes for birthdays and special occasions and a biscuit with the odd cup of tea not a couple every time you put the kettle on. You may consider healthy alternatives such as Date Loaf or Bran Muffins in the recipe section of Harry's Healthy Hints.

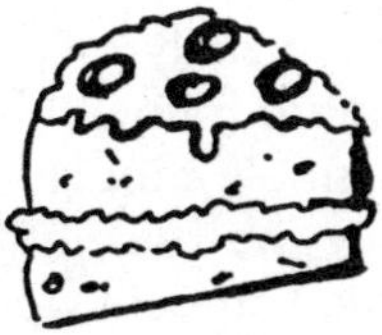

A fellow was explaining to me why his six cream biscuits each day was probably *not* the reason why he was overweight. As he spoke I discretely tapped the keys of my calculator. When he had finished the explanation I politely told him that he therefore ate 2190 every year, which was 883 000 kilojoules and that if he wanted to burn it off in a single walk he would have to walk from Sydney to Canberra and back. He agreed that the small things can add up quite quickly.

Note: 'Biscuits' also include savoury and cracker biscuits — keep them for parties. Prefer low fat varieties such as Ryvita, Crackerbread and so on.

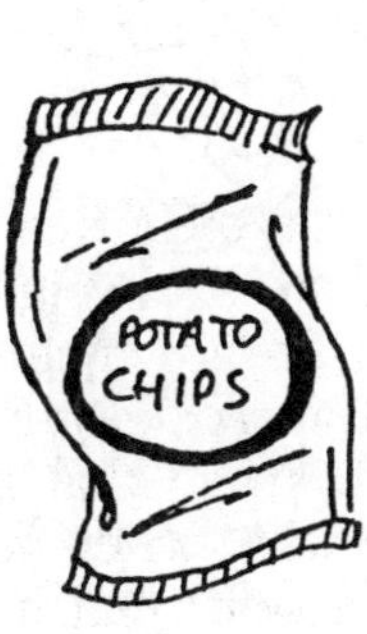

16. AVOID fatty snack foods. Avoid chocolates, potato crisps, corn chips and so on. Have alternatives available. Some snack foods such as chocolate also contain large amounts of sugar.

For the 'choc-a-holic':
If you truly love chocolate it is unlikely you will successfully give it up completely, nor do you need to. Please follow this advice. Once every week go and buy a small chocolate (no more than six normal squares), buy the best, eat it, enjoy it and don't feel guilty. This small amount won't make much difference to your weight loss effort. Then when you are finished tell yourself 'That's all until next week'. If you do this you may satisfy the craving for chocolate which will threaten your whole effort.

Carob is not the healthy alternative it is made out to be. Sure it has not the caffeine of chocolate but it has almost as much fat. Again go for the real thing and enjoy it only as a treat.

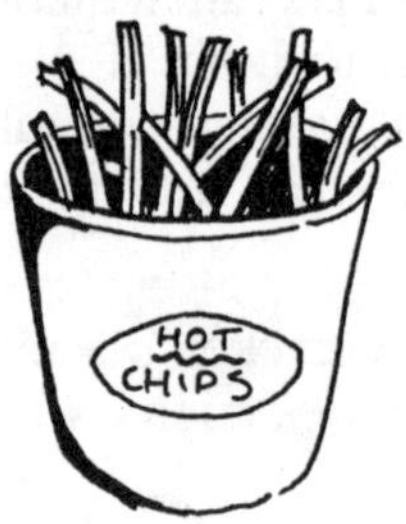

17. AVOID fatty take-aways. Pies, sausage rolls, fried chicken, fried fish and chips and pizza are best avoided. When you buy these foods there is usually a healthy alternative, such as a sandwich, that is just as accessible. As well as adding large amounts of fat, therefore energy, to your diet, they often contain large amounts of salt.

Low fat cooking

There are three places where you make decisions regarding whether you eat low fat or otherwise:

- the shop — the starting point;
- the mouth — the obvious final test;
- the kitchen — the sometimes forgotten important go-between.

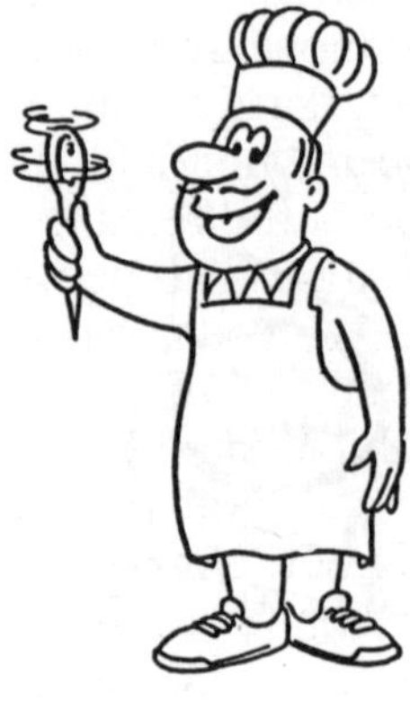

What you do in the kitchen is very important. Foods that are high fat such as pork chops can be modified by removing the fat to leave a piece of meat that fits well into your Good Eating Guidelines. The opposite occurs when you buy low fat ingredients such as potatoes but add fat or oil during the cooking process by making french fries. Your cooking methods will play a major role in determining whether or not the food you eat is truly low fat.

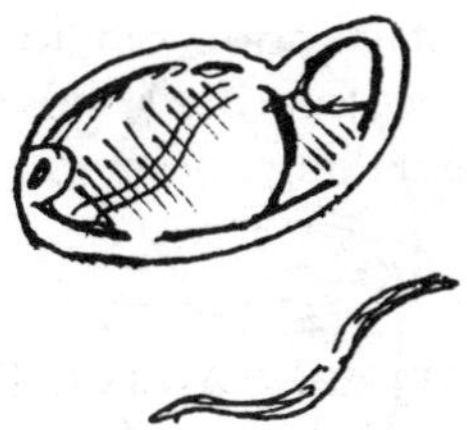

LOW FAT COOKING GUIDELINES

18. DO trim the fat from meat BEFORE cooking. Take your time and remove as much visible fat from the raw meat as possible. The small amount of fat that remains tends to cook out of the meat.

19. DO skin and remove fat from chicken BEFORE cooking. It is important you do this before cooking because most of the fat on a chicken is in the skin or just under it. Removing the skin has a two-fold effect. Firstly you are removing a large amount of fat directly. Secondly some of the remaining fat will cook out rather than being held in by the skin. For your own interest place the skinned chicken beside the fat and skin you have removed, it is surprising just how much fat commercial chickens contain.

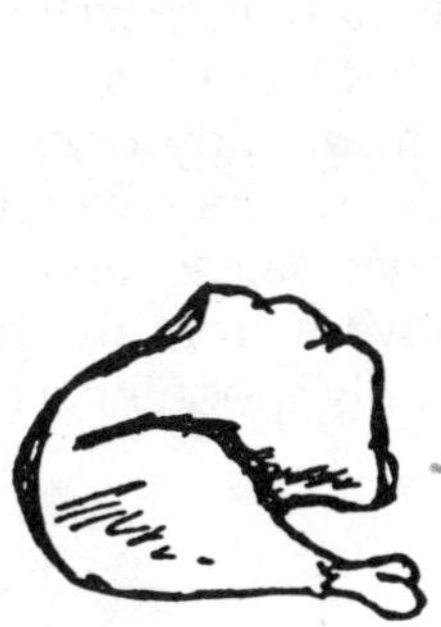

If you have not skinned chicken in the past you may find your first couple of experiences a little trying. Persevere. It will only be a short time before skinning chickens is a routine part of your cooking. Try using kitchen scissors.

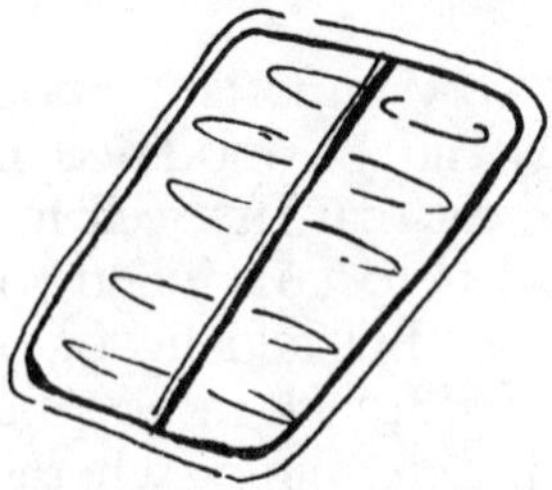

20. DO grill or roast foods rather than pan frying. Roasting and grilling allows fat to cook out of the meat where frying tends to cook fat into it. Using a rack insures the fat moves away. Dry frying is OK if you have been particular about trimming fat before cooking.

21. DO allow homemade soups, stews and casseroles to cool, then remove the hard layer of fat. Remove fat from pan juices before making gravy. If you have not done this in the past you may be surprised at the amount of hidden fat in your meals. Ideally you should prepare these types of meals a day early and leave them overnight. The hard fat layer that forms can be easily removed. Preparing the meal early does require some planning but these types of dishes improve their flavour when left to stand. If you haven't planned ahead and have not the time to let the dish cool, remove it from the heat and let it sit for five minutes before carefully spooning as much liquid fat away as you can.

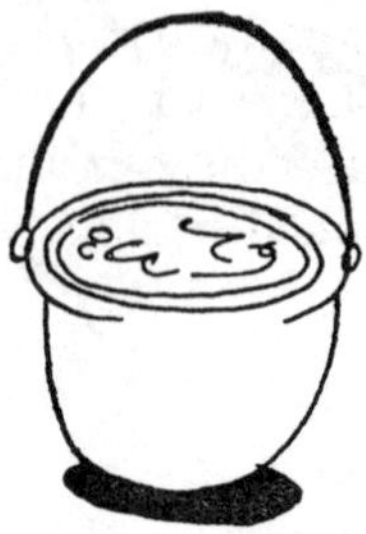

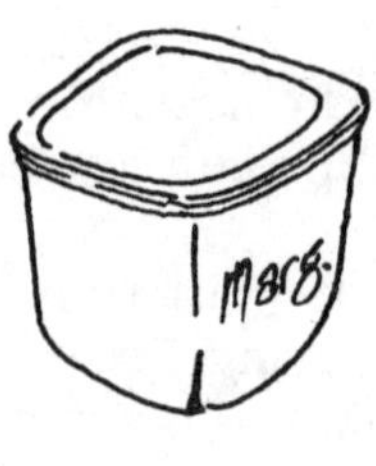

22. LIMIT fats and oils in the preparation of food. Limit the number of dishes you prepare that require oil in the cooking process. If a dish does require oil be as sparing as possible . If a recipe says a tablespoon you can probably do the job just as well with a teaspoon.

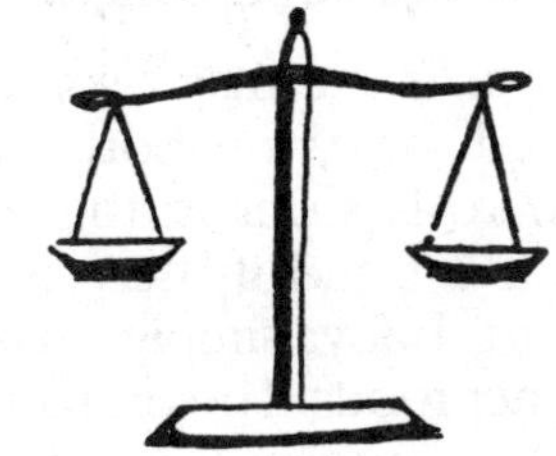

23. LIMIT the amount of meat and chicken you eat. Stick to 90 to 140 g per day. Weigh the meat or chicken before cooking. Do this several times so you can reasonably estimate the quantities in the future without the need for scales. Buy your meat in these quantities. For example if there are four people for dinner buy 500 g of meat.

This may be one of your most important guidelines and if you are a big meat eater you may find it a little difficult to adjust. You will need to add something new to the plate to compensate for the smaller meat portion. Don't simply increase the amount of the same vegetables, this may make your meal boring. See Harry's Healthy Hints section for some ideas.

What about eggs?
Eggs are relatively low in fat but are often limited because they have a high level of cholesterol. If your cholesterol is normal four to five eggs per week is not a problem. If your cholesterol is elevated limit eggs to two to three per week.

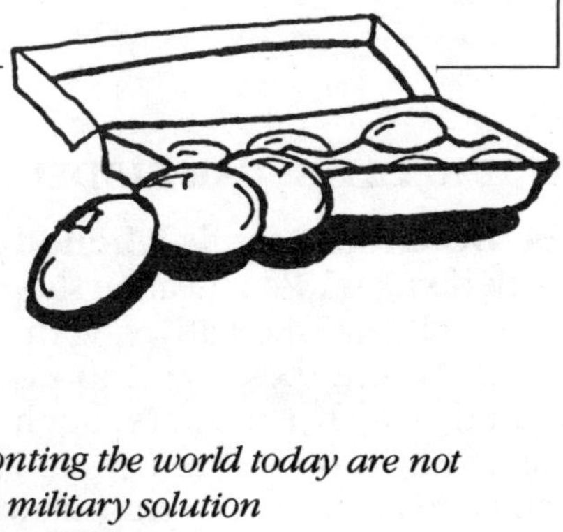

The basic problems confronting the world today are not susceptible to military solution
JOHN F. KENNEDY

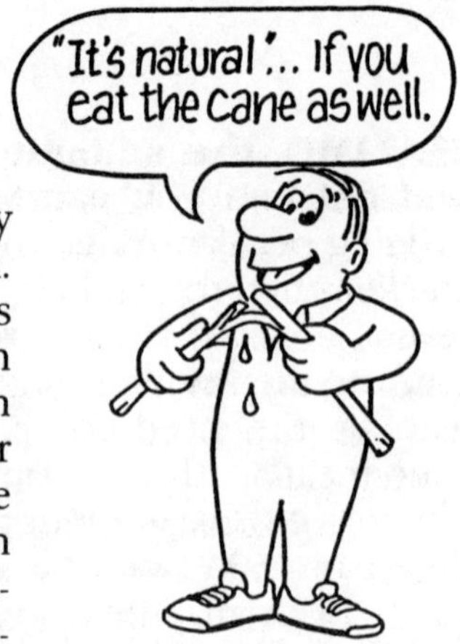

Eating less sugar

Sugar is the major source of energy used by your body to function. There is sugar in the natural foods you eat and if there is not enough your body simply makes it from other foods. The problem with sugar is that humans learned how to refine it and then put it in foods in a much higher concentration than it naturally occurs. For most of human existence the only concentrated form of sugar was wild honey. In those days you would have had to endure considerable pain to earn the sweet treat and most of us would have considered it not worth the effort.

Sugar in concentrated forms such as white, brown or raw sugar or in chocolate, soft drinks, biscuits and so on can provide more energy than your body needs. Your body doesn't simply discard this excess sugar energy, but switches on a very important survival mechanism and converts it to body fat. This survival mechanism has been vital for our existence because in the past we would fatten up in the times of plenty and use the fat to survive when food was scarce. This survival mechanism is now having the reverse effect. In our modern Western society few encounter times when food is scarce. If we are not careful, we just keep putting the weight on. The result is poor health such as heart disease.

EATING LESS SUGAR GUIDELINES

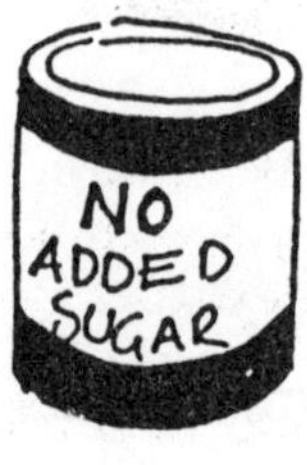

24. DO choose foods labelled 'no added sugar'. Be a healthy shopper and seek out alternatives with less sugar. Where possible choose no added sugar products such as canned fruit packed in natural juice rather than in heavy syrup or fruit-only jams.

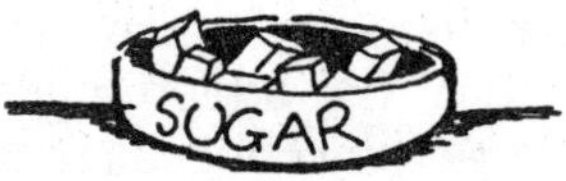

25. AVOID adding sugar to food or drinks. If you have been a sugar lover for years you may find this guideline a little difficult. If so cut down gradually, aiming not to be adding sugar in two months. You may like to use artificial sweeteners instead.

Try adding fresh, dried or stewed fruits to cereals and other foods you normally add sugar to. In cooking use healthy cookbooks that only use small amounts of sugar or none at all. You may be surprised at the sugar-free treats you can make.

'But wait! Can I have just a little bit?' If you feel that completely going without sugar is too tough, limit yourself to four level teaspoons per day. Remember that it is the first thing to go if your weight doesn't keep moving toward its ideal target.

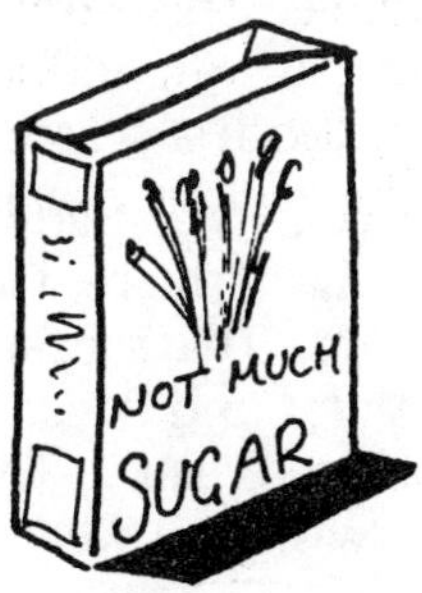

26. AVOID breakfast cereals which contain lots of sugar. If a breakfast cereal tastes very sweet it probably contains a large amount of sugar — choose another brand. Some cereals contain only small amounts of added sugar and are OK — let your taste be the judge. Read labels carefully and if sugar is high on the list of ingredients avoid that brand.

Be aware that sugar comes in different forms; for example, a common Australian muesli has sugar, raw sugar, honey, dextrose. Don't be tricked, it's all sugar. Choose cereals that are based on whole grains such as wheat biscuits, puffed wheat and rice, rolled oats and natural muesli with little or no added sugar. Try Quick and Easy Muesli in the recipe section.

27. AVOID jams, honey, syrups, and confectionery. Rather than thick jam on toast every morning save it for a Sunday morning treat or try 'no added sugar' jams or choose another alternative. Have sweets only sometimes when they are offered to you, don't have an open packet in the car.

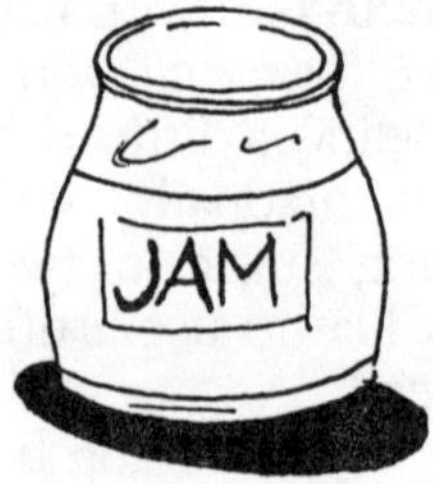

28. AVOID soft drinks and cordials which contain sugar. Soft drinks contain as much as 12 teaspoons of sugar per can. That means lots of unwanted energy which can become unwanted fat. It is very difficult to lose weight if you regularly drink soft drinks and cordials. Try artificially sweetened soft drinks or choose something altogether different such as plain old water, straight or with a dash of lemon.

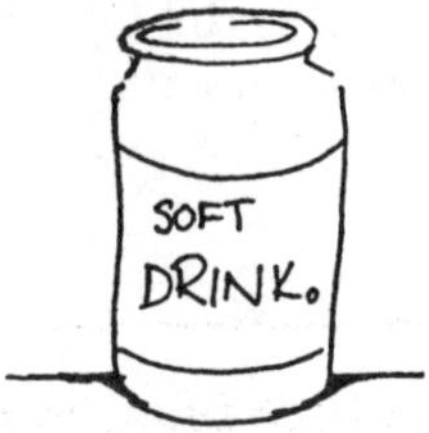

'THAT'S EASY...'

I was delivering a seminar to a group of people who had high cholesterol. As I concluded a session dealing with the Good Eating Guidelines a fellow stood up and said, 'That's easy! — all I have to do is invent a high fibre, low fat and sugar-free food that tastes like chocolate, cheese and ice cream'. (Thank you David Price for the classic comment. I wish you well with the invention.)

Leaving salt until another day, this concludes your Good Eating Guidelines. Go back and reread your Healthy Eater's Creed and pay particular attention to the phrase 'Slow, steady and forever'. The Good Eating Guidelines may mean significant changes to your diet but take your time, don't rush it. Remember, you are the driver on this journey so you choose the pace that best suits you.

- ☐ *Review the Good Eating Guidelines Check List (Chart 2) to make sure you have highlighted all the guidelines relevant to you.*
- ☐ *Each week go to Chart 2 and tick the guidelines you are conforming to.*
- ☐ *Make an appointment to work through the chapter 'Increase Activity' — approximately 15 minutes.*

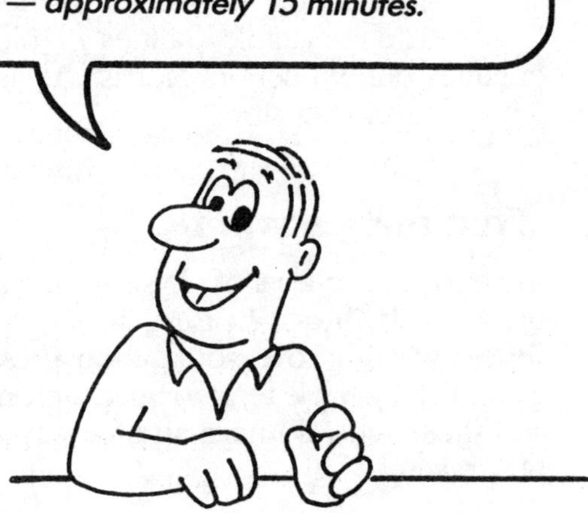

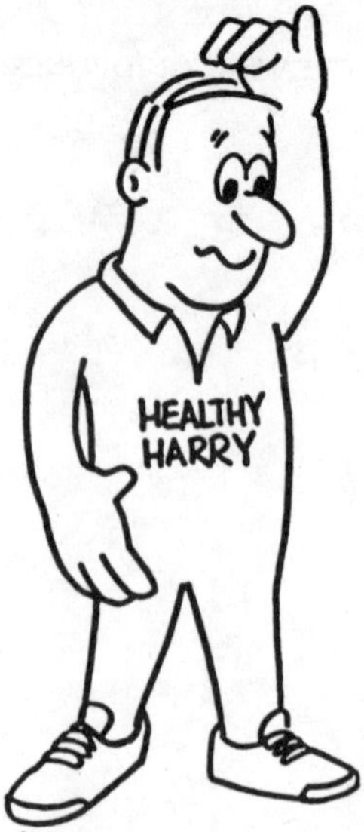

Increase Activity

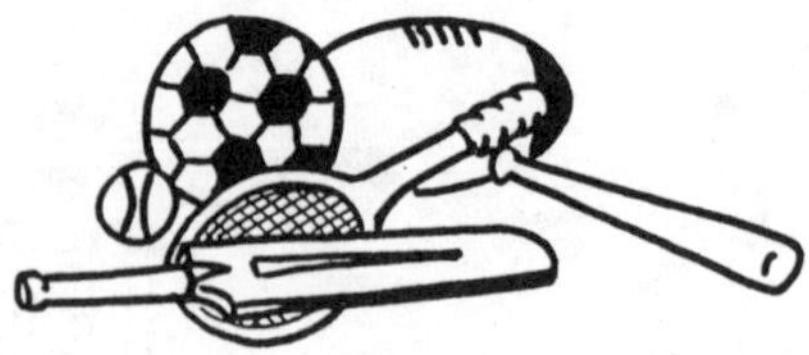

'Never Ever Stop'

Mrs Ethel Morris (102 years) has reached her remarkable age without the discomfort of any significant illness. She attributes her healthy longevity to being committed firmly to her lifelong motto: 'Never ever Stop'. That meant walking, walking and more walking. Whether it was to the shops, visiting friends, the races (which she particularly enjoyed) or for the sheer pleasure of it, Mrs Morris walked.

Testimony to her resolve was the fate of her antique rocking chair. The chair spent its life in a dormant state gathering dust. A relative suggested to Mrs Morris that she curb her physical activity and retire to the more typical image of a granny in a rocking chair. The rocking chair was swung smartly into action — straight to the nearest charity auction.

The inevitable frailties of old age have become her enemies but, while Mrs Morris has any say in the matter, she will — never ever stop.

What makes you fit?

Increasing your level of physical activity will improve your level of physical fitness. In turn, increasing your level of physical fitness will improve your blood pressure and your health in general. Fit people tend to be less prone to having heart attacks and those who do have an attack have a much better chance of surviving.

As well as directly improving blood pressure, regular physical activity can have powerful indirect effects. Firstly, if you exercise regularly you burn up more energy which means you can tilt your energy balance in favour of weight loss. Secondly, regular exercise is one of the most powerful tools you can employ to relax. Exercise doesn't fix the cause of stress but it does help you cope with it much better. You are able to think more clearly which means more astute decisions regarding your health.

Get FITT

To achieve the most from your exercise program you need to apply the FITT guidelines: **F**requency
Intensity
Time
Type

- **Frequency.** The minimum number of exercise sessions per week is four. It's ideal to get some exercise nearly every day.
- **Intensity.** As a general rule the exercise needs to make you puff a little and maybe, raise a light sweat. This is brisk exercise. You should be able to talk comfortably to someone who is exercising with you. If you are unable to comfortably hold a conversation you are probably exercising too hard (or you are swimming!) so ease back a little.
- **Time.** Each exercise session should last at least 15 minutes though 30 to 60 minutes is ideal.
- **Type.** The exercise needs to be aerobic which simply means that it increases your heart rate. See 'Pick an Activity' (page 59) for some suggestions.

Those who think they have no time for bodily exercise will sooner or later find time for illness
EARL OF DERBY, 1873

Exercise Heart Rates:
Often when authors are advising on the intensity at which people should exercise they use the phrase — Exercise Heart Rate Zone. It is a suggested range that your heart rate (pulse) should increase to when you are exercising in order to achieve a fitness effect. This program is not suggesting Exercise Heart Rate Zones for two reasons:

- if you are not accurate when taking your pulse you may act on an incorrect recording and over exert yourself;
- many blood pressure medications affect heart rate and conventional exercise heart rate zones may be dangerously high.

If you want to take your pulse as a means of monitoring exercise intensity ask your doctor or a health professional who has a background in prescribing exercise programs for people with high blood pressure. Have someone else take your pulse twice to confirm your accuracy.

Enjoyment is the key

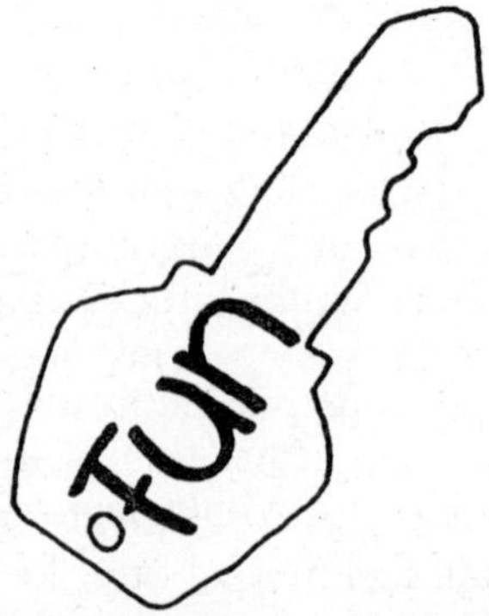

Choose activities that you enjoy and will be likely to keep doing for a long time. If you become bored with a particular activity find another rather than stopping exercise altogether. Variety and other people help increase the enjoyment you get from exercise and this in turn keeps you motivated.

Give plenty of thought to your selection of fitness activities to insure that you settle on a program that best suits you. You may need several activities to keep you interested or you may prefer a single activity that fits your busy schedule.

A cardiac patient for whom I was designing a rehabilitation program was very easily satisfied. After recovering well from his heart attack his doctor suggested he walk four kilometres every day. He chose not to walk around the neighbourhood, as would have been expected, but rather around his living room. It was a large living room but still required 150 laps to travel the 4 km. He probably has to replace his carpet on a regular basis but he is quite happy with his program. It provides him with the exercise he needs. His program is right for him.

You have to choose a program that conforms to the FITT guidelines and is right for you. You may be the opposite to this particular gentleman and may choose a different activity every day — that's your decision.

Pick an activity

Read the following list of aerobic activities and select an exercise program that will best suit your lifestyle. After reading the list you will complete My Exercise Program in the Record Section.

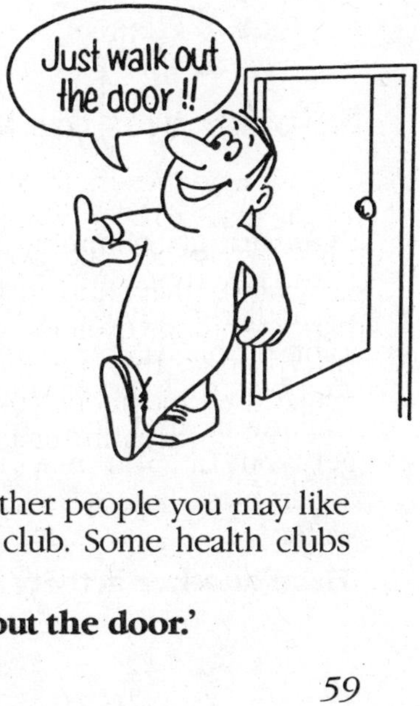

Walking. Regular brisk walking improves and maintains fitness. It's the cheapest, easiest and most accessible exercise for most people. It's so simple — all you have to do is walk out the door and come back a short while later. Walking is also a great way to relax and may be a good time to discuss things with someone. Why not substitute a half hour walk for a television show — you'll feel much better for it.

If you enjoy exercising with other people you may like to join a bushwalking or orienteers' club. Some health clubs have formal walking classes.

'It's simple — just walk out the door.'

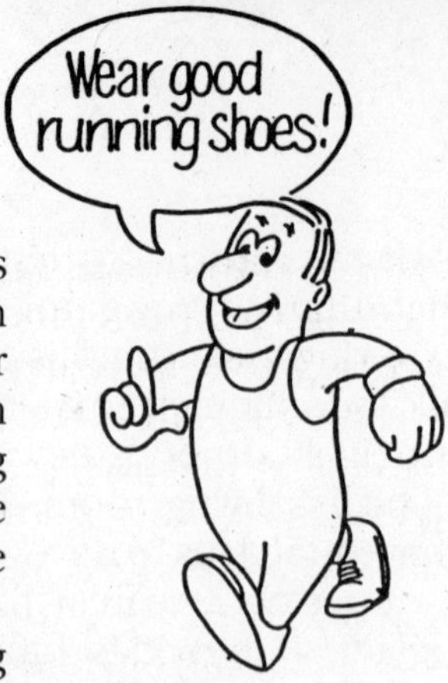

Jogging. Jogging is a great fitness activity if you enjoy it and are in shape for it. If you are not a regular jogger and want to be, start with short easy jogs in your walking program and gradually increase the jogging time while reducing the walking time.

If you are more than 8 kg heavier than your ideal weight don't start jogging until you have lost some weight. If you have back pain or other joint problems it may be wise for you to choose another activity.

'Be sure to wear good running shoes.'

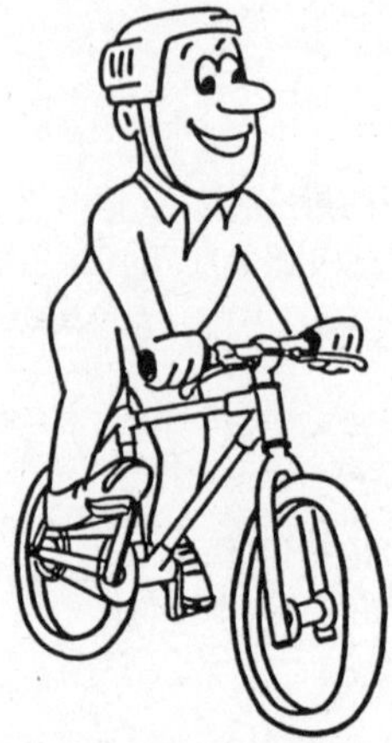

Cycling. Cycling is a great activity for improving and maintaining your fitness. Start at an easy pace and build up gradually. Provided you keep away from bumpy roads, cycling is good exercise if you have a back problem.

'Safety first — wear a helmet.'

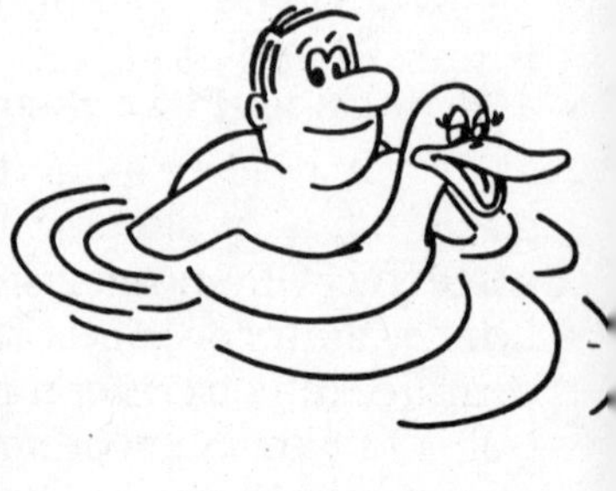

Swimming. Swimming is a useful fitness activity for most people, particularly anyone with back or joint problems, because the water supports their body weight. Simply walking up and down the pool will get you fit. You may like to try aquarobics classes — aerobics in water.

'Have another activity ready to go as soon as it gets too cold to swim.'

Tennis, Badminton, Table Tennis. Singles is great for fitness whereas doubles is only moderately so. If you are in a group that plays only doubles try to arrange a 15 to 30 minute hit of singles with someone during the session.

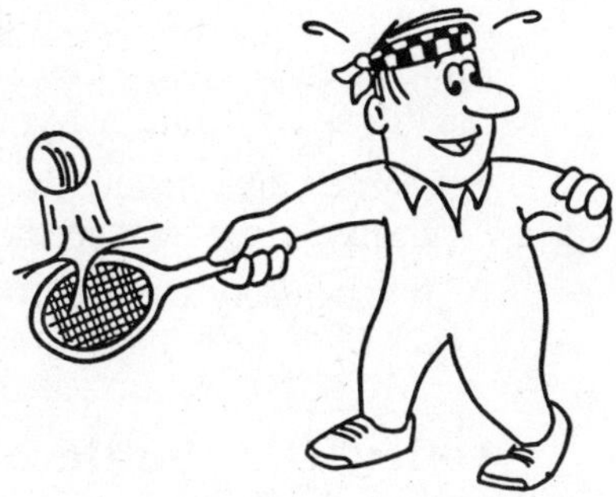

These activities require other people which means a little more organising at first but it has the advantage of someone else to encourage you in the times where you may otherwise have let the session slip by.

You will be surprised at the fitness benefit you can get from table tennis, so if there is a table that has been resting for years in your shed, dust it off and get into action.

'It takes a few games to pick up the skills — stick at it, the fun will follow.'

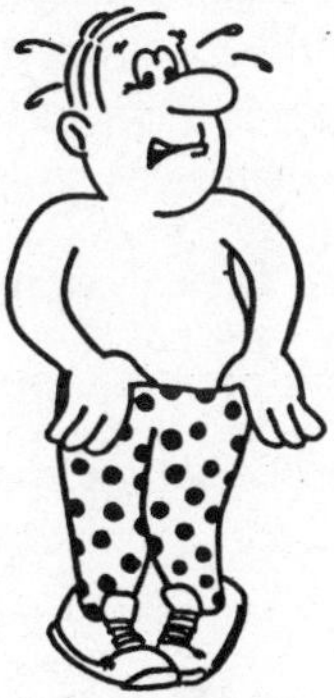

Aerobics classes. Aerobics classes are great fitness activities if you choose a class that is suitable for you. Don't try to keep up if the class is too vigorous. If you have back problems or are more than 8 kg above your ideal weight choose low impact classes.

'How do you like Harry's new leotards?'

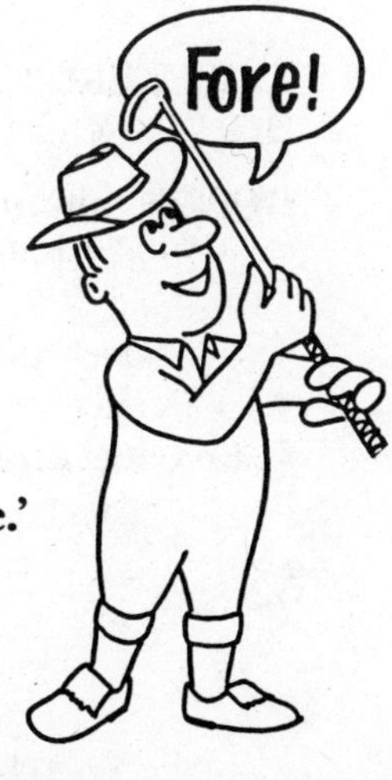

Golf. Golf is only of moderate fitness value because of its stop-start nature. You can rely on golf for some of your fitness program but choose another activity to top up your exercise requirements.

'Don't stay too long at the nineteenth hole.'

Football, basketball, hockey, touch footy, indoor cricket. These activities are great for fitness *but* you must already have a reasonable level of fitness and train for your sport on a regular basis.

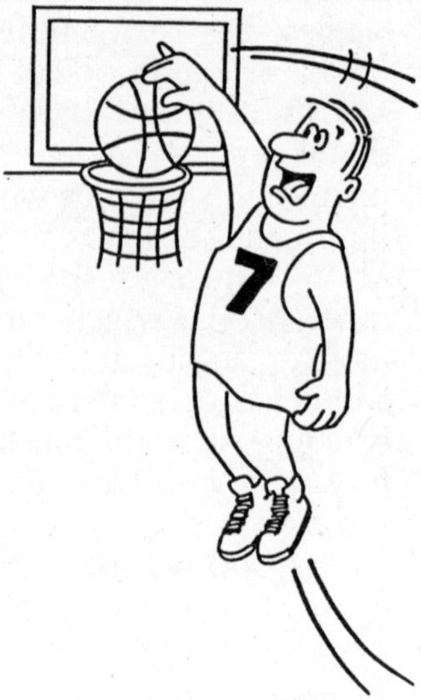

'Exercising in a team helps you stay committed.'

Volleyball, shuttlecock, hit a tennis ball against a wall, play ball with a friend. It doesn't matter what you do as long as you are getting a little puffed doing it. That can be as simple as hitting a tennis ball against a wall or buying a cheap shuttlecock set from the supermarket — you don't even need the net. See how many times you can hit the shuttlecock back and forth without hitting the ground. It won't be long before you get a sweat up.

'You don't need expensive equipment or fancy venues to get fit. Be imaginative and practical.'

'Another good reducing exercise consists of placing of both hands against the table edge and pushing back.
ROBERT QUILLEN

THE EXERCISE DON'TS

DON'T exercise if you are ill.

DON'T continue exercise if you:

- feel pain or tightness in your chest, neck, left arm or jaw.
- become breathless without over exerting yourself.
- have palpitations.
- feel dizzy, ill or black out.

If you have any of these experiences see your doctor.

DON'T over-do it.

DON'T exercise within one hour of a heavy meal.

DON'T exercise in very hot weather. Wait until the cool part of the day.

DON'T do vigorous exercise without stretching and warming up first.

- ☐ *Complete My Physical Activity Program on page 138. Also make your first entry in your Physical Activity Diary on the same page. For the next 20 weeks you will make daily entries into your Diary.*
- ☐ *Make an appointment to complete the next chapter 'Not Too Much Grog'. It will take about 10 minutes to complete.*

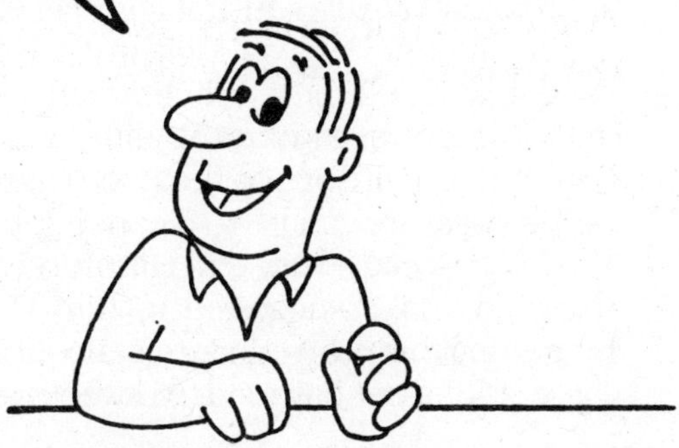

Not Too Much Grog

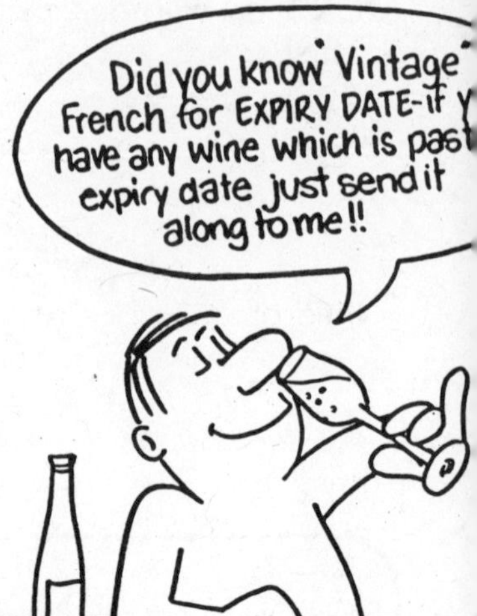
Did you know Vintage
French for EXPIRY DATE-if y
have any wine which is past
expiry date just send it
along to me!!

Some researchers claim that small amounts of alcohol may have a cardio-protective effect — it may guard against heart disease. I am not certain whether or not they are correct but I sure have my fingers crossed. What I am certain of is that beyond a certain amount, alcohol has devastating effects on health. In excess alcohol can shoot blood pressure up to very high levels, it raises blood triglycerides (a fatty substance in the blood which, in excess, may contribute to the development of heart disease), it causes liver disease, heart disease and other diseases as well as many social problems. Alcohol accounts for the premature death of approximately 4000 Australians every year.

Alcohol is also high in food energy so contributes to weight gain and therefore indirectly effects blood pressure.

Alcohol can be the difference between people having high blood pressure or not. Joe is an example of how sensitive blood pressure can be to alcohol. Joe was drinking six to eight alcoholic drinks every day. His blood pressure is usually greater than 150/105. I suggested to him that we do an experiment by getting him to reduce his alcohol consumption to two or three drinks per day for a two week period. I closely monitored his blood pressure during this time. Two days after the experiment began his blood pressure was on borderline high, around 145/95. It remained at this level until two days after he resumed his normal level of drinking. It only took two days for the alcohol to increase his blood pressure back to dangerously high levels.

It is a major challenge for health professionals to advise on levels of alcohol consumption. On one hand consideration has to be given to widespread social use of alcohol and to the fact that there is little evidence that low levels of consumption is harmful to health. On the other hand consideration must be given to the devastating effects alcohol can have on health if consumed in excess. I believe Harry's Rule of Twos is a reasonable response to the challenge. It is simply applying the SELF Test to alcohol.

A man is drunk when he feels sophisticated but can't pronounce it
W.G. PLUNKETT

Harry's Rule of Twos

- **Two** a day is plenty
- **Two** AFDs (Alcohol Free Days) a week
- **Two x twos** is a treat
- **Two** treats is too many

Sorry! You can't save the Twos up for one big party at the end of the week.

Harry's Rule of Twos refers to standard drinks, see page 124.

- Two a day is reasonable.
- Two Alcohol Free Days each week tends to break the habit forming effect of alcohol that can make it such a demon.
- Two x twos (4 drinks) is a treat in that once a week you can have a few drinks without going overboard. But you shouldn't have two treats in a week.

Here is a sample week that fits Harry's Rule of Twos.

Sunday	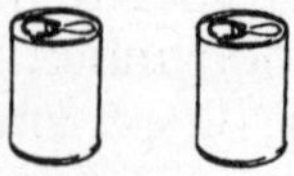	You might have a couple of beers after working in the garden or while watching the football
Monday	AFD	A good day to have an Alcohol Free Day
Tuesday	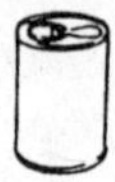	A drink before dinner
Wednesday	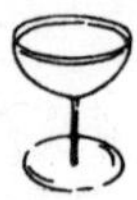	A wine or two with dinner
Thursday	AFD	Another AFD
Friday	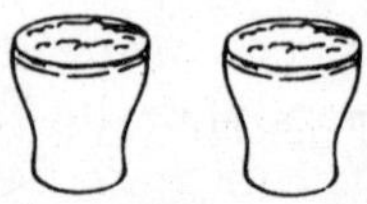	A stop at the pub on the way home from work, two's plenty
Saturday	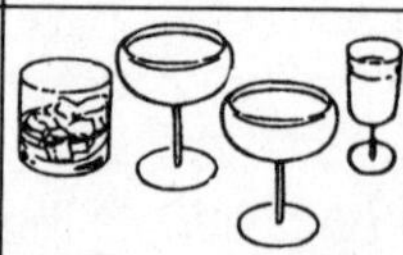	You're out to dinner and four drinks is a treat. More than one treat in the week is too many

If you are a heavy drinker — six or more drinks per day — you may find Harry's Rule of Twos too difficult to achieve at this stage. Considering the nature of alcohol this is understandable. Attempt to reduce your consumption by half. Later you may find it easier to adopt Harry's Rule of Twos.

If you find cutting down your alcohol consumption very difficult you can seek help. This is not as frightening as it seems. You don't have to make a fuss about it, just have a chat with your doctor and he or she may direct you to professionals in this field. Alternatively many workplaces now have confidential alcohol counselling programs to help you put alcohol back into its right perspective. Or you can call organisations such as Alcoholics Anonymous.

If you feel you need help — go and seek it. Yes, it can be hard to admit to someone else (and even more so to yourself) that you have a problem with alcohol. Just the same you must bite the bullet and do something. It's a small but extremely valuable investment in your future health and happiness.

Putting off an easy thing makes it hard, putting off a hard thing makes it impossible
W.G. PLUNKETT

What do I drink instead?

Cutting down on alcohol certainly does not mean cutting down on your social life. If you stop your social life you are probably not making the program fit your lifestyle. You need to have alternatives. Consider these:

- **Good old water.** It has been our most popular drink for the past two million years. Have it straight or flavour it with lemon juice, orange juice or low joule cordial. If you have normal cordials, be sparing. If you are hesitant about the quality of your tap water you may consider purchasing a water filter. They are becoming very common and many are relatively inexpensive.
- **Soda water.** By itself or flavoured, it is a sparkling alternative. Try it with bitters or non-alcoholic mixers such as Claytons, but be sparing with those that contain sugar.
- **Mineral water.** Most brands are fine though some have high salt levels. If you drink mineral water check the bottle for sodium content. If it is less than 15 mg per 100 mL it's OK.
- **Low joule soft drink.** Limit normal soft drinks as they have too much energy.

- **Fruit juice.** Limit to one or two glasses per day. Try having half juice with half soda or mineral water.
- **Reduced alcohol drinks.** If you choose reduced alcohol beers (2.0 to 2.5% alcohol), Harry's Rule of Twos becomes the 'Rule of Threes', and a treat is six drinks. If you choose half nips of spirits or mix wine half-and-half with soda or mineral water, the 'Rule of Fours' applies, and a treat is eight drinks.

Hints to make your task easier

- Drive to the place where you will be drinking. This is the most socially acceptable excuse for knocking back a drink.
- On your shout buy a non-alcoholic drink.
- Don't allow your glass to be filled until it's empty.
- If you think your friends are going to give you a hard time because you choose non-alcoholic drinks simply tell them you are fixing your blood pressure and fewer drinks sure is better than pushing up daisies.
- Challenge your friends to join you. Behind those beer glasses lies a potential walking group or tennis team.

The driver is safer when the road is dry. The road is safer when the driver is dry
W.G. PLUNKETT

- ☐ *Record your daily alcohol consumption in Chart 6 'Harry's Rule of Twos' in the Record Section.*
- ☐ *If you are a smoker read through the chapter 'No More Smokes'.*
- ☐ *Make an appointment to work through the chapter 'Relax' — approximately 15 minutes.*

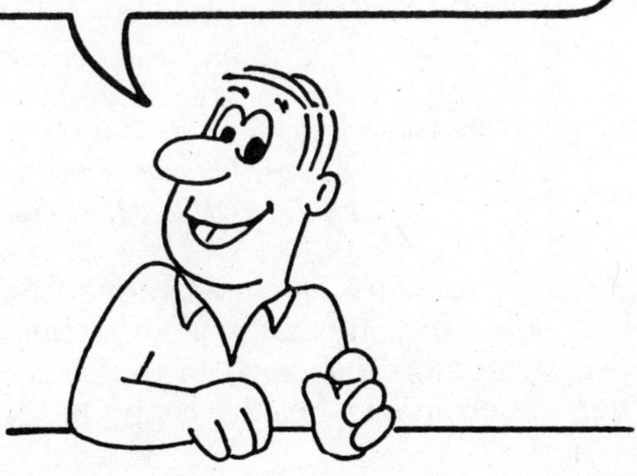

No More Smokes

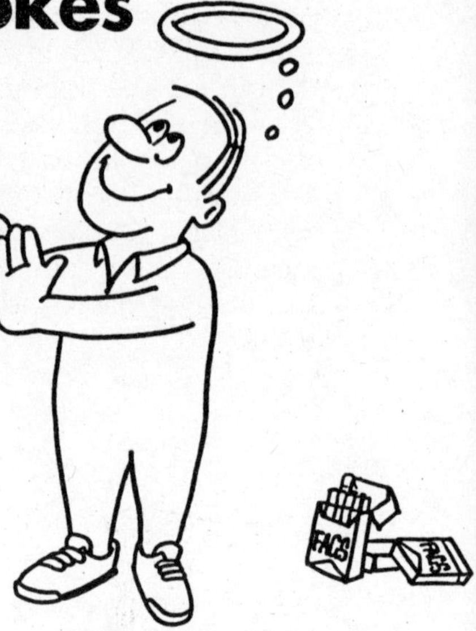

'The World Health Organisation rates cigarette smoking as the major cause of premature death in Western society'; 'The health department claims 16 000 Australians die from smoking each year;' and on and on and on it goes. You've heard these types of comments a million times before, but although there is little doubt about the truth of these statements, this is probably not what you really want to hear again. What you want to know is 'How the hell can I kick this habit without going 'round the bend or breaking the bathroom scales in two months time.' Unfortunately this program is unable to offer a magic answer. It would if it could but there simply isn't one. It's a tough job to kick the habit but one you can and must succeed at.

Have you ever noticed how much gets done when you say the words 'I can't'
HEALTH YOURSELF NEWSLETTER

There are many and varied methods of quitting. The best one is the one that works for you. The following method is a suggestion that may do the trick. Carefully follow each step to becoming a healthy, happy and confident non-smoker.

1. Record your cigarette consumption. The first job in your long preparation for the big day is to record approximately how many cigarettes you smoke each day. Do this by updating Chart 5 'Quit Check List', daily. Many people who record their cigarette consumption become tuned in to their habit and tend to smoke less.

QUIT CHECK LIST

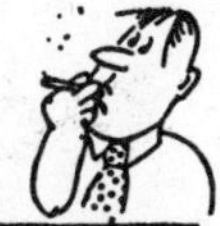

On the ___/___/___ I begin my new life as a healthy, happy and confident non-smoker.

	Sun	Mon	Tue	Wed	Thur	Fri	Sat	Total
Week 1								
Week 2								
Week 3								
Week 4								
Week 5								
Week 6								
Week 7								
Week 8								
Week 9								
I am a healthy, happy & confident non-smoker.								
Week 10								
Week 11								
Week 12								
Week 13								
Week 14								
Week 15								
Week 16								
Week 17								
Week 18								
Week 19								
Week 20								

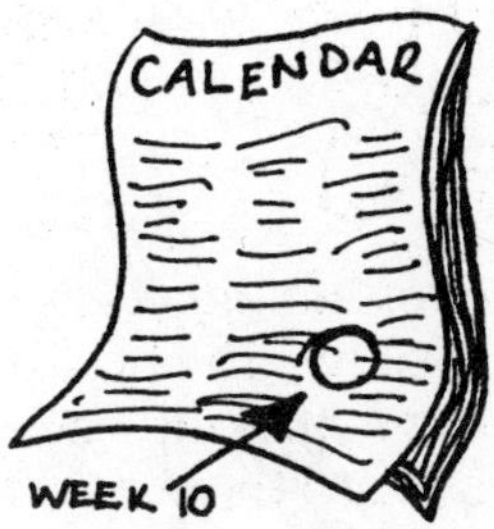

2. Set a quitting date. Your Quit Check List has a space provided to write in your proposed quitting day. Select the Saturday before Week 10.

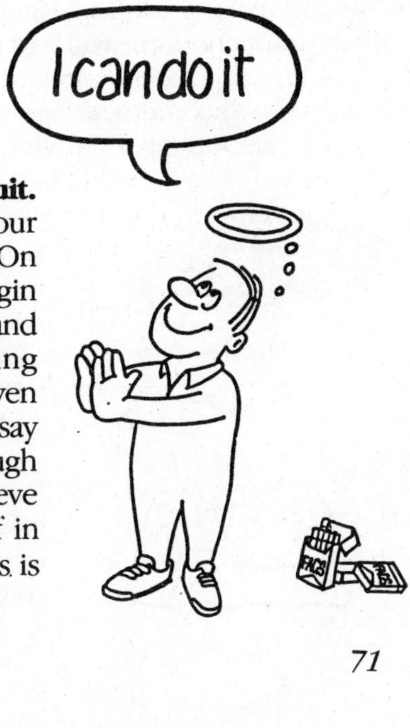

3. Believe you are going to quit. Each time you make an entry in your Quit Check List read the words 'On the ________________ (date) I begin my new life as a healthy, happy and confident non-smoker.' Reading these words is simple and may even seem a little childish but if you say it often enough and with enough conviction you will start to believe it. Armed with a genuine belief in yourself your potential for success is virtually unlimited.

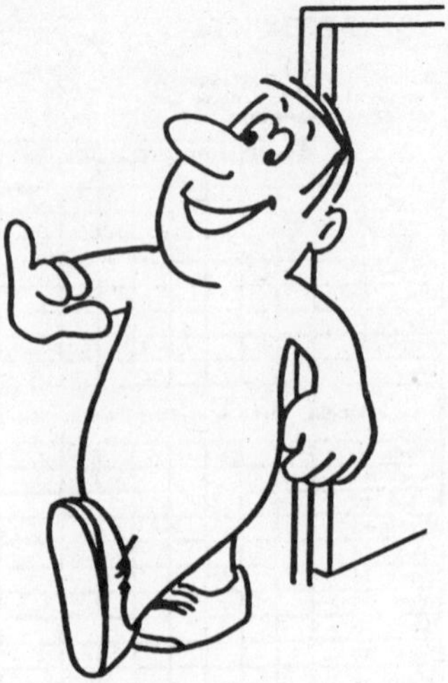

4. Be physically prepared. One of the reasons for setting your quitting date later in the program is so that you are physically prepared. You will be leaner, fitter and feeling much better about yourself which will make quitting much easier. You will have also adopted the Good Eating Guidelines that will reduce the possibility of you picking at high energy foods which could cause you to put on weight. Weight gain is the fear of many who are quitting.

5. Quit and celebrate. When the big day arrives — quit. This should be one of the proudest days of your life so don't let it quietly slip by, make a fuss. Celebrate by really treating yourself. Invite other people to join with you in the celebration. You are making one the most important decisions you will ever make and that's no exaggeration.
Buy yourself something special with the money you will be saving.

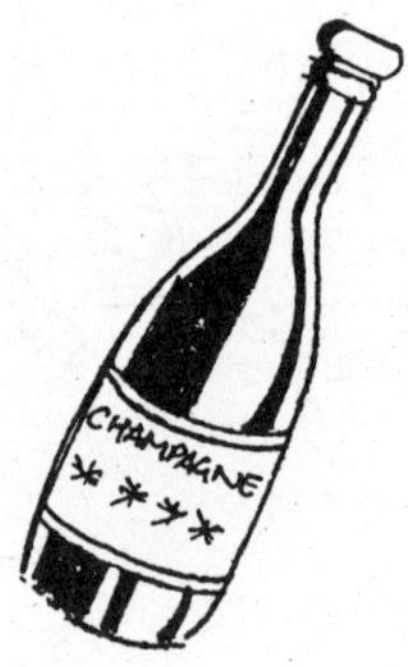

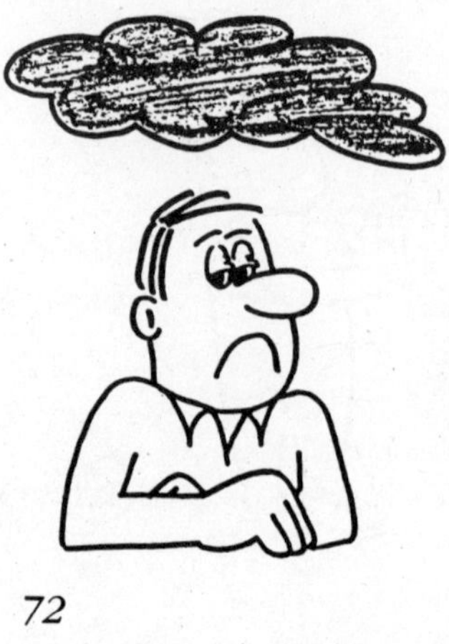

6. Weather the storm. The first two weeks are tough going. It would be silly to pretend they are going to be easy. Accept that it is tough but keep telling yourself you have got this far and you're not turning back. It will get easier.
Each day you enter that magic 'zero' in your Quit Check List repeat the words — 'I am a happy, healthy and confident non-smoker'.

Hints to help you weather the storm:

- Ask all those near to you to be tolerant because you may be a bit grumpy for a while.
- Have non-fattening nibbles available because you will be reaching for something. Try strawberries, dried fruit or nuts (not too many), celery or carrot sticks. Chew gum if it satisfies you.
- As much as possible avoid situations where you will be tempted to break out. Ask the people you know who smoke not to smoke near you and not to offer you a cigarette.
- Increase your exercise program. This will help relieve the frustrations.
- Take extra 'time outs' (see 'Relax' chapter) at work so you can plan each period of work to insure you can cope without reaching for the cigarette packet.

7. Keep at it. If you do break out it's just a setback, certainly not a failure. You must keep trying because your life really does depend upon it.

Don't fail for want of trying, give it a go
W.G. PLUNKETT

Ease Back on Salt

'Ease Back on Salt' has been deliberately left to Week 6 because:

- eating less salt is usually less important than weight loss in the management of high blood pressure;
- your salt consumption has probably already reduced as a result of adopting the Good Eating Guidelines to lose weight;
- to restrict salt at the same time you are making changes to lose weight may have overloaded the program in the early stages.

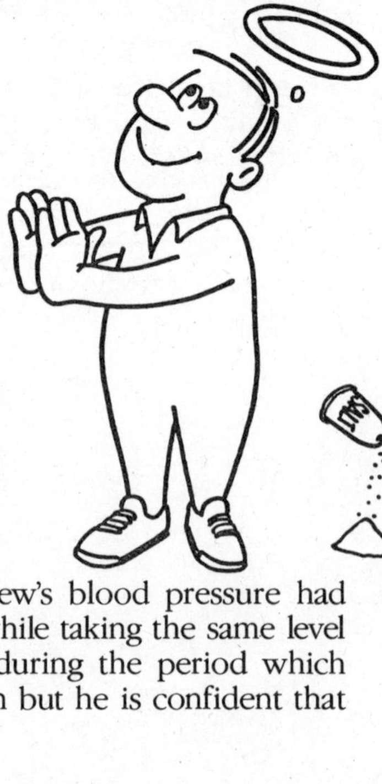

Salt restriction has been proved to reduce blood pressure in some people. Lew is one such example. Lew has a natural tendency to have high blood pressure. He is a non-drinker, non-smoker, very fit, appears to manage stress well and is within his normal weight range. He consumed a moderate amount of salt. During mid 1987 Lew's blood pressure was 161/92 (126 recordings) while taking medication (50 mg Capoten daily). Lew decided to embark on a strict salt reduction diet in an effort to improve the situation.

In the later part of 1987 Lew's blood pressure had improved, 143/85 (98 recordings) while taking the same level of medication. Lew did lose 2 kg during the period which may have made a small contribution but he is confident that salt restriction played a major role.

EASE BACK ON SALT GUIDELINES
Highlight the guidelines that are relevant to you. Also highlight them in your Good Eating Guidelines Check List.

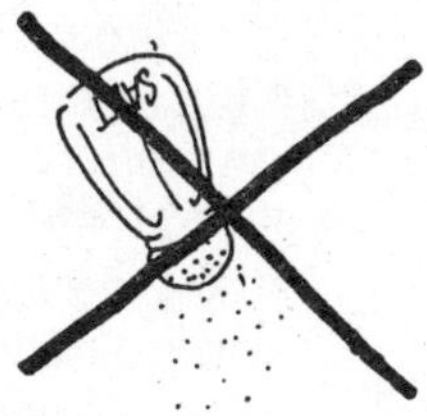

29. AVOID adding salt at the table. This may be difficult if you have been adding salt to your food for as long as you can remember. Cut down gradually and aim not to be adding salt to your meals in six weeks' time.

'Salt craving' is acquired by habit and is not your body telling you it needs salt. In a few weeks your craving for salt will fade and your taste will become more appreciative of the natural flavours of food.

Try alternatives such as pepper, herbs, lemon juice or vinegar. Salt substitutes such as potassium salts are fine but if you have a heart or kidney condition check with your doctor first. Be careful when buying salt substitutes as you may be buying ordinary salt in disguise such as herb salt or natural sea salt. Some lite salts have the amount of ordinary salt reduced. You may find them helpful while you are cutting down.

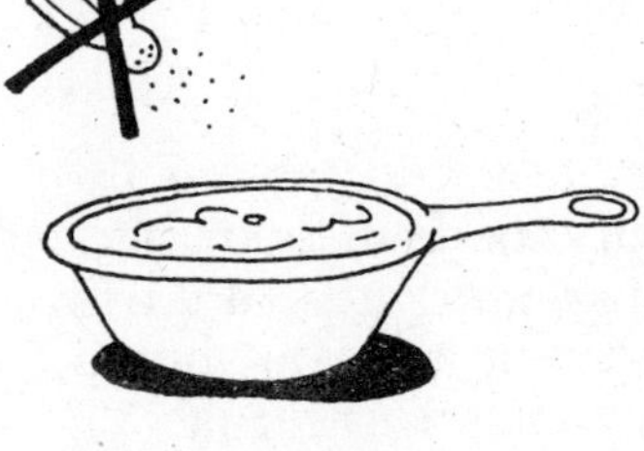

30. AVOID adding salt to cooking. Again it is wise to cut down gradually. Pepper, herbs, spices, curry, wine, lemon juice or vinegar will help boost the flavour of your cooking in the absence of salt.

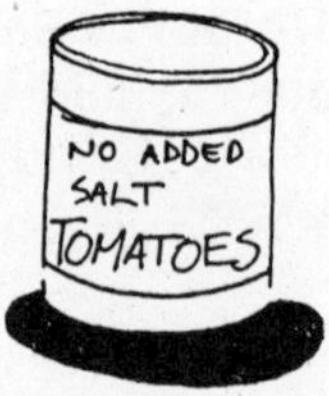

31. PREFER 'no added salt', 'low salt' or 'reduced salt' products. In response to health conscious shoppers, supermarkets carry a large range of products with less salt. Where possible buy these products. For example:

- Low salt bread is a wise choice considering ordinary bread has a medium salt content and is eaten in relatively plentiful quantities in a healthy diet. Try a few different brands to find one you enjoy. If, after several attempts you still find low salt bread unpalatable return to normal bread and concentrate on other areas to reduce your salt intake.
- Choose salmon in water rather than in brine.
- Many canned foods have no added salt alternatives. You may be surprised at how different they taste. This is testimony to the large amount of salt that is used in the processing of many foods.
- Low salt or salt-free margarine and butter are readily available

Reduced salt products are better than the regular products but still may contain a considerable amount of salt and are best used sparingly.

Do the best you can:
For example, let's say you are unable to buy salmon packed in water (no added salt) — don't do without, buy it packed in brine but drain it well. A can of red kidney beans has a lot of salt so rinse them before using, and so on.

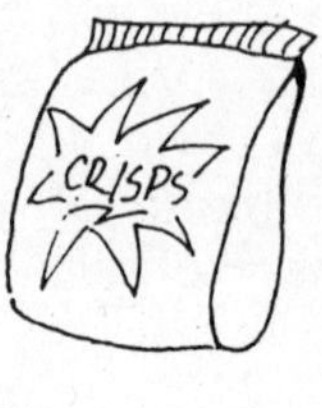

32. LIMIT salty foods. If food tastes salty then you can be sure that it has a high salt content and you should limit it. See 'Where's the Salt'.

The following lists indicate the amount of salt contained in different foods. When reading the lists keep in mind that it may not be foods in the very high group that are contributing most salt to your diet, as you often eat less of these foods. For example you may spread only 3 g of vegemite on your toast but eat 50 g of cornflakes in a serve.

WHERE'S THE SALT?

VERY HIGH GROUP	HIGH GROUP
salts (garlic, herb or sea salts) **meat tenderisers** **MSG** **stock cubes** **corned beef** **ham** **olives** **salted fish** **meat extracts** **yeast extracts (Vegemite)** **gravy powder** **soy sauce and** **most bottled sauces** **some take-away foods** **parmesan and blue cheese** **many snack foods**	bread margarine fried take-aways canned and packet soups cracker biscuits Chinese foods Lebanese food devon chicken loaf pâté potato chips pizza hard cheeses/cheese spread canned fish pies, sausage rolls many breakfast cereals
MEDIUM GROUP	**LOW GROUP**
sweet biscuits many breakfast cereals canned vegetables cheese cake cottage cheese cakes pastry many sweets	**grains** **fresh or frozen vegetables** **dried beans and dried fruit** **ricotta cheese** **eggs** **meat** **fish** **herbs** **bran** **unsalted nuts** **foods labelled 'no added salt'**

Relax

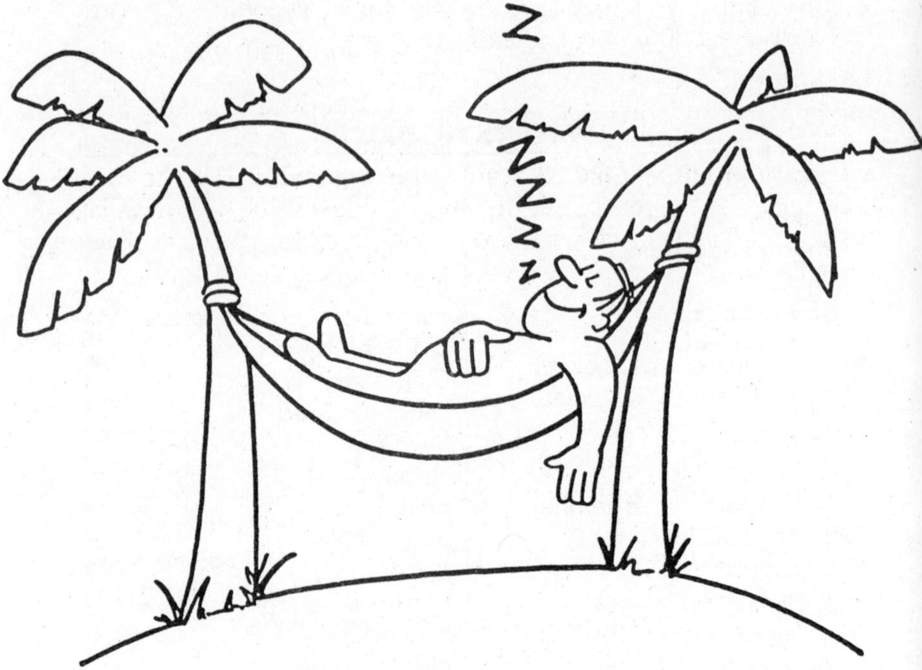

Tom held a very high responsibility position, only ten people in Australia were licensed to do his particular job. He was exposed to a high level of work stress. For many years he was a very effective stress manager and conducted his work with enjoyment and efficiency. In early 1990 the pressures of work and life in general increased. At the same time Tom's ability to manage stress lessened. It lessened to the point where he almost allowed stress to devastate his life.

As Tom's ability to manage stress diminished his physical condition also deteriorated. He became quite overweight, his fitness level was very low and he was drinking more than he normally would. Tom's health progressively deteriorated until one day he collapsed at work . His medical advisers suggested that it would be too risky for him to remain in his position and he would have to continue in a less responsible role at work. Indeed this was a correct decision but it created another source of stress for Tom to cope with and at this stage he was coping very poorly with any stressful situation.

A full medical check up revealed that he had high blood pressure and small changes on his electrocardiograph (heart monitor) that indicated the possibility that he was developing heart disease. That was the last thing Tom wanted to hear. Tom was allowing even minor stressful events to upset him. In Tom's own words he was 'a mess' and didn't care whether he 'lived or died'.

One of Tom's work associates suggested he give our centre a call and get into shape and maybe this would help him cope with life a little better. Tom thought he had nothing to lose so he decided to 'give it a go'. He was in such a nervous state that he sat and literally watched the telephone for 20 minutes before mustering the courage to make the phone call to book an appointment. Here is a man who has, for years, been making extremely important decisions on a daily basis.

If you worry about yesterday's failures,
then today's successes will be few
ANON

Tom's story had a happy ending. In a relatively short time he had lost 15 kg, vastly improved his fitness level and was drinking well within Harry's Rule of Twos. His blood pressure had returned to normal without the need for medication. The suspicious changes on his electrocardiograph were no longer present which could possibly be a direct result of his actions. He was coping well enough to begin confidently the review process prior to resuming his old job. Most of all he was again happy. He was winning the prize that for some time had been eluding him — *quality of life.*

What caused Tom's high blood pressure? Was it stress? No, I doubt it very much and most health professionals would agree with me. The blood pressure changes were most probably a direct result of being overweight and very unfit. There is very little research evidence that links stress directly with large and sustained elevations in blood pressure (contrary to what most people in the community are lead to believe). But stress caused Tom to neglect his health. If he had remained an effective stress manager he would not have allowed his physical condition to deteriorate as it did. Stress really did cause his blood pressure to rise — indirectly.

If you are not managing stress well you are less likely to make astute decisions regarding your health in general. For example, the person who is not coping with work stress is more likely to work back late, hurry home, grab a pizza and a six pack of beer for dinner, then sit back in an armchair explaining why there is no time in the day for exercise. People who are not coping with stress are more likely to be smokers, comfort eaters or 'hit the bottle'. Good stress managers make better health decisions.

Stress is a more complex issue than other health parameters such as fitness or smoking. For this reason many people don't tackle the issue of stress and leave it in the too hard basket. This program does not attempt to analyse stress or to give all the answers to individual stress problems. It provides you with real tools to help you become a more effective stress manager and to relax. Things you can *do* — remember the program is all about *doing* the things you can to improve your health. Indeed there are many great books written about stress and I recommend you read them *but* only after you have devoted time to doing the simple things you can do to relax.

Stress is not something that happens around you — stress is *your reaction* to what is happening around you.

A worry is only a worry — if you worry about it
HEALTH YOURSELF NEWSLETTER

Stress management tool box

Here are tools people use to manage stress and relax:

- **The way I think.** The way you think determines what you are and what you do. If you keep thinking you are a great stress manager you will start to move in that direction. You will enjoy life more and get more out of it. This may sound a little distant from reality but it isn't. In fact the way you think is the most powerful influence in your life — *think* about it.

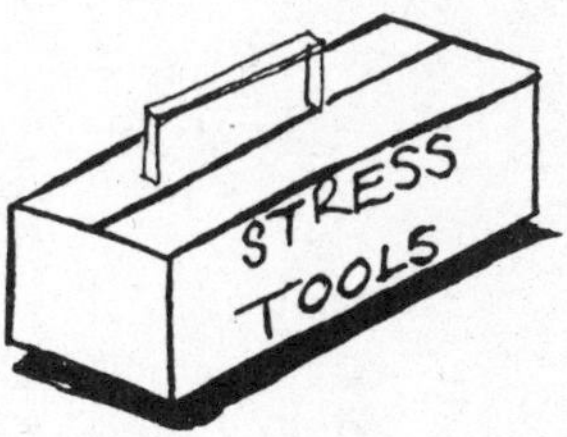

  'The Way I Think' Affirmations. This will assist you to tune your mind into believing you are a relaxed, effective stress manager. You have already started by involving yourself in this program. You are probably already feeling better about yourself because of the positive lifestyle change you are making.
- **Physical exercise.** Exercise is a powerful relaxation tool. When you exercise, your muscles do real work and then they relax. Your mind clears. Exercise also promotes a more restful sleep which may improve your mood, work performance and general coping ability. How do you feel when you finish an exercise session?
- **Time outs.** These are explained later in this chapter.
- **Formal programs.** There are many valuable courses available in the community that may help you become a better stress manager. For example, straight out stress management programs, grief management, programs to improve work efficiency or to improve communication skills and so on. These are great but make sure you are doing the above three points as well.
- **See a psychologist or a counsellor.** This course of action is reserved for those having considerable

difficulty in managing stress. If this is you don't be afraid to seek professional help.

- **Massage, yoga, tai chi, meditation, biofeedback.** Many people find these activities perfect for relaxation. Try them and see what works for you.
- **Do a 'just for the fun of it' activity at least once each week.** What's stopping you from getting up one morning and packing a picnic basket with fruit and sandwiches or cereal and milk and going to a pleasant place, preferably near nature, for breakfast. A park or the beach would be nice — you know a place. You may have a swim before you eat. After breakfast go for a long walk. Then sit back and relax. Tension just drains away. Or what about a movie, a drive in the country, a swim in the surf, read a book, or whatever it is you really enjoy doing? It's hard to be nervous and tense when you are happy, smiling and having fun.

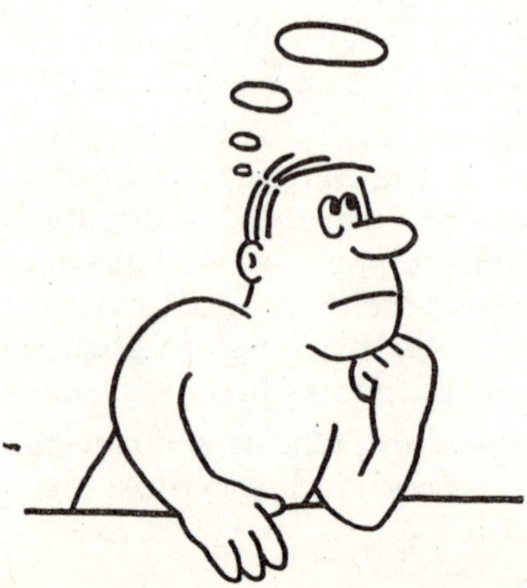

'The Way I Think' Affirmations:

Here are eight positive affirmations that will help you to grow to believe you are a relaxed person and effective stress manager. If you firmly commit yourself to these affirmations you will move in their direction. Read these affirmations and feel them on a daily basis. Take three long, slow and deep breaths before you begin.

- Stress is not something that happens around me. Stress is *my reaction* to these happenings. I have control over my ability to manage stress.
- I take reasonable action to modify the happenings that cause me to react in a stressful fashion. When I am unable to modify these happenings I simply accept them.
- I do not get unduly upset by my mistakes. After all, I am only human.
- I devote my energies to *now* rather than worrying about what might have been or what might happen in the future.
- I am strong at saying *No* when I mean *No.*
- I am an organised person who sets priorities and gets things done.
- I am a caring and worthwhile person. I really do like myself — I really do!
- I *smile often.* In fact I am smiling at this very moment.

Keep cool and collect
MAE WEST

Time outs

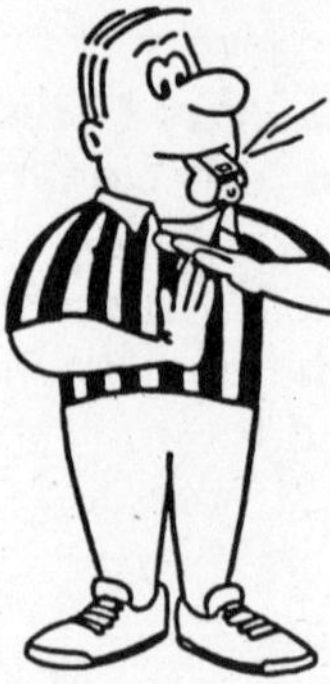

Imagine a game of professional basketball. Five players determined to have the ball at one end of the court and another five just as determined to have it at the other end. The result is continuous frantic activity. Players are running this way and that yelling to each other; referees are working up a sweat trying to keep things under control while being yelled at by almost everyone in the stadium, coaches look like their blood pressure is so high they are about to explode and the crowd is screaming for its heroes to succeed. Suddenly the referee blows his whistle and calls, 'Time out'.

The tempo completely changes. Players move to the side of the court to catch their breath, referees have a chat, coaches, well, they try to look calm and the crowd relaxes back in their seats. During the time out everyone settles down and readies themselves for the next part of the game.

Your daily life can be like a basketball game, full of continuous frantic activity. Unfortunately many people forget to blow the whistle and call 'time out'. They don't take short deliberate breaks to have a rest and gather their thoughts before embarking on the next stage of their busy day.

You are going to start blowing your imaginary whistle and take some time outs, two every day. Give yourself two ten minute breaks every day to have a brief rest from your activities and regather your thoughts. Time outs are deliberate periods of time away from what you are doing. You might take the phone off the hook and rest back in your chair or go for a walk around the block or pull off the road in the heavy traffic to look at a pleasant scene or read a book or meditate and so on. Whatever it is you do, it must be a clear break from your daily activities. Time outs are an appropriate time to read your 'The Way I Think' Affirmations.

Be able to be alone. Lose not the advantage of solitude
SIR THOMAS BROWN

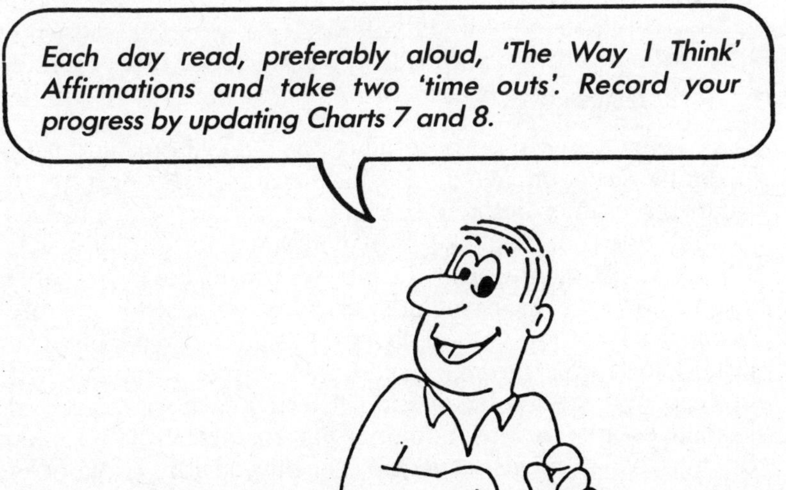
Each day read, preferably aloud, 'The Way I Think' Affirmations and take two 'time outs'. Record your progress by updating Charts 7 and 8.

Harry's Healthy Hints and Recipes

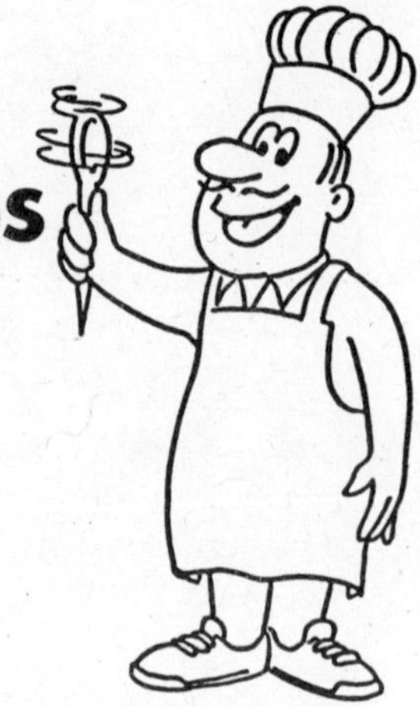

Most recipe books become dust collectors on book shelves. They are dusted off when special treats are needed or in the case of healthy cookbooks when someone gets a pang of guilt about their health.

Before opening a healthy cookbook, this one included, set yourself a mission. Let's say most Tuesday evenings you prepare braised chops, vegetables and chips. After applying your Good Eating Guidelines you have decided the meal is too fatty and you want a replacement. Your mission is to find a healthy replacement for this meal. Your mission has the following conditions:

- the healthy meal will not cost significantly more;
- the healthy meal will not take much longer to shop for or to prepare, though on the first occasion it may, simply because it's different;
- the healthy meal will easily slot into your usual routine;
- it tastes good.

Now you can purposefully open a cookbook and make a definite selection. When you have made a selection, try it two or three times before discarding it. Make as many changes (healthy ones) as you like so it will suit your cooking style and taste. After the third time you will have probably transferred the recipe to memory and it will be a second nature choice. This recipe section is not designed as a complete cookbook. It is a starter kit of simple to prepare meals that you can use as replacements. There are also suggested alternatives for various cooking ingredients. If you enjoy cooking special meals I suggest you buy healthy cookbooks and have fun brewing up some gastronomic storms.

THE ALTERNATIVES	
NOT SO HEALTHY	HEALTHY
sausages, fatty chops, fatty mince meat	lean meats, low fat sausages (if you can find the genuine article), chops from which you can easily remove the fat
pies, sausage rolls, pasties, deep fried chicken, potato scallops, fish and chips	wholemeal sandwiches or rolls; pita bread with filling; Homemade Pizza (see recipe section); tacos made with beans; barbecued chicken is OK if you remove the skin and visible fat; hamburgers with salad and wholemeal roll are not too bad
biscuits, cakes, sweet pastries, cream buns	fruit breads, muffins or healthy recipe cakes. Try Bran Muffins or Date Loaf (see recipe section)
chocolate, confectionery, crisps	dried fruit, fresh fruit, nuts (maximum a small handful each day), no added sugar health bars
high fat cheeses	low fat hard cheese, ricotta or cottage cheese
sweet desserts such as ice cream, custard made with whole milk, apple pie and cream and so on	fresh, stewed or canned fruit with Strawberry Cream or a variation, (see recipe section); custard made with skim milk, try Vanilla Rice Pudding in the recipe section
sweet cream	blend ricotta cheese with vanilla and a little milk
sour cream	low fat natural yoghurt alone or blended with ricotta cheese, add a little vinegar if you like a sharper taste
high fat mayonnaise	base mayonnaise on condensed skim milk or low fat yoghurt, try Mayonnaise (see recipe section)

Everyone has experienced French onion dip, cabanossi pieces, cheese cubes and crackers when they have walked into a party — not very healthy. Try some of these healthy suggestions and listen to the positive feedback you'll get.

HEALTHY ENTERTAINING	
NOT SO HEALTHY	HEALTHY
cabanossi salami full cream dips salted crackers party pies sausage rolls crisps corn chips pretzels confectionery salted nuts cheese platters olives cocktail frankfurts	fruit platters: try rockmelon sliced in a fan, small bunches of grapes, piles of strawberries and raspberries, halved passionfruit, coconut dipped banana pieces, kiwi fruit, orange segments, lychees, sultanas or dried fruit healthy dips based on ricotta or cottage cheese — see recipe section for chilli, crab, French onion and corn flavoured dips for dippers use vegetable pieces such as celery, carrot sticks, green beans, cauliflower and broccoli flowerettes, try also bread sticks or lightly toasted wedges of pita, Lebanese or plain breads serve bowls of cherry tomatoes, cherries, unsalted nuts (be sparing), sultanas, raisins, dates, dried fruits such as apricots, apples and pears popcorn small wholemeal sandwiches

Meal suggestions

The old adage 'Breakfast like a king, lunch like a queen and dine like a pauper' is very good advice. Generally in our community we get it around the other way by starting the day with a small breakfast or skipping it all together. Then a small lunch followed by a large dinner. It's unreasonable to expect people to revert fully back to the old adage but the following suggestions will help you move in that direction.

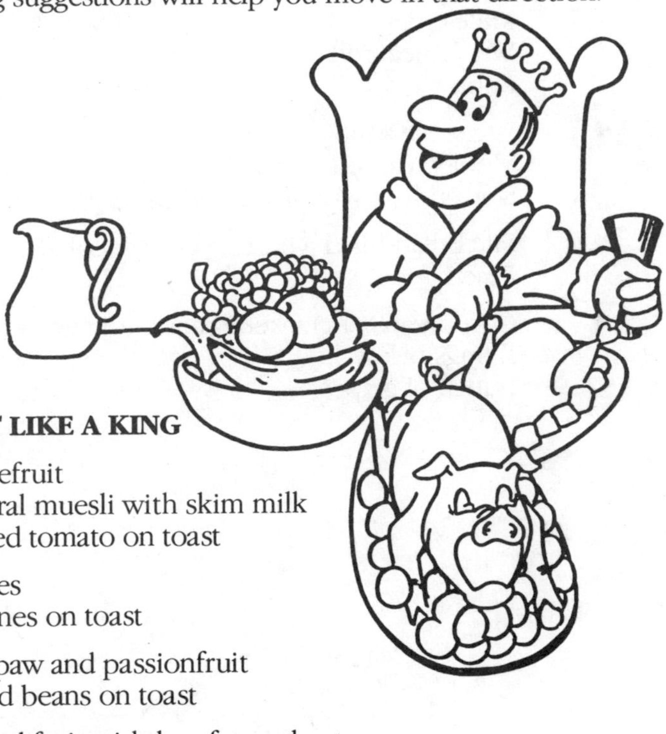

BREAKFAST LIKE A KING

- Grapefruit
  Natural muesli with skim milk
  Grilled tomato on toast
- Prunes
  Sardines on toast
- Paw paw and passionfruit
  Baked beans on toast
- Stewed fruit with low fat yoghurt
  Asparagus on toast
- Fresh strawberries or a slice of rockmelon
  Rolled oats with skim milk
  Simmered tomato and onion on toast
- Banana or orange
  Wholegrain cereal with skim milk
  Grilled cottage cheese and sliced tomato on toast
- Slice of pineapple
  Wholegrain wheat biscuits with skim milk and sliced banana
  Scrambled eggs on toast

LUNCH LIKE A QUEEN

- Tuna or salmon salad
  Orange
- Minestrone
  Wholemeal roll
  Apple
- Vegetable soup
  Wholemeal roll
  Stewed fruit with low fat yoghurt
- Pita bread filled with rice or bean salad
  Peach
- Crispbreads or crackerbreads with any of the sandwich fillings below
  Bunch of grapes

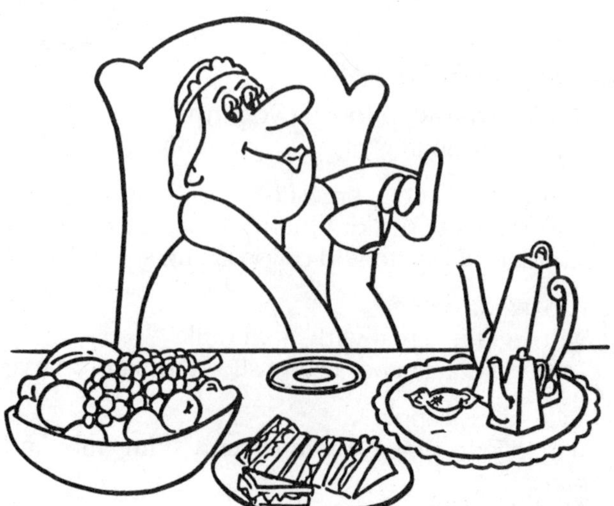

- Sandwiches — take your pick — put these fillings on wholemeal bread, crispbreads, bread rolls or fill pita or Lebanese pockets:
  - tuna and green salad vegetables
  - mixed bean salad and ricotta cheese
  - lean smoked turkey with asparagus
  - grated carrot, sultanas and walnuts
  - cottage cheese, apple and celery
  - lean chicken and salad
  - ricotta cheese, tomato and capsicum
  - banana and cinnamon
  - mushroom, coleslaw and sprouts
  - lean beef, mustard, grated zucchini and radish
- Leftovers, leftovers and more leftovers — if you have prepared a healthy meal for dinner it will still be healthy the next day so have it for lunch. This is certainly better than grabbing an unhealthy lunch on the run. It also has the bonus that you won't have as many second helpings for dinner if you know you are leaving some for tomorrow's lunch.

DINE LIKE A PAUPER
(Well, not too poor)

See recipe section for details

- Spaghetti Bolognaise
- Whole Chicken in Vegetable Sauce
- Fillets in Foil
- Minestrone
- Veal and Chickpea Casserole
- Annette's Tropical Chicken
- Homemade Pizza

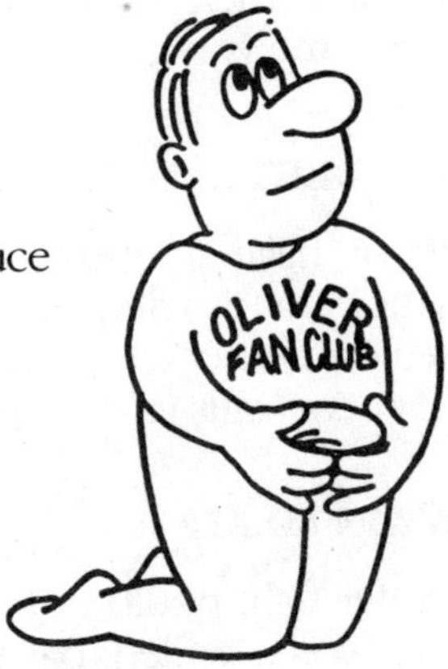

Dining out

A client, Allan, said to me that he was happy with his new healthy lifestyle but for one thing. He told me that he and his wife would look forward to their once a month treat — a special meal at the Hilton. They had not had their special treat since Allan had his heart attack many months ago. My response was immediate: 'Go and have your special meal two weeks in a row to catch up'. You see Allan forgot to apply the SELF Test to his dining out. The changes that really counted for Allan were that he was now using about one-third the margarine that he previously used, he was eating leaner and less meat and was drinking less alcohol. It's the everyday things that make the difference. Treats are fine if they are kept as treats.

If you dine out once per month or less my advice is 'Go for it': eat what you want, have the treat and don't feel guilty.

If you eat out two or three times per month you can still treat yourself but you need to be a little prudent with regard to the type and quantity of food you order.

If you eat out once or more per week you have to be extra careful. Restaurants usually present larger meals than you would normally eat and they are often high in fat. Be very selective and *ask ask ask*! Don't be afraid to ask for your meal to be prepared in a way that suits you. Almost always the restaurant will be happy to cater for your requests because you are their valued customer. Consider the following hints next time you go out to dinner.

ENTREES

If you have an entree avoid dessert or vice versa. Avoid cream sauces and fried foods. Prefer fresh oysters, other fresh seafoods (not too many prawns if your cholesterol is elevated), fruit cocktails and vinaigrettes.

MAIN MEALS

Prefer fish, poultry (leave the skin) and lean meats. Look for the words grilled, baked or steamed. Steer clear of words like creamed, cream sauce, cheese sauce, fried, pan fried, sautéed, butter sauce, basted and hollandaise.

When ordering a grilled dish ask for it to be grilled without fat. Suggest that they instead use wine or lemon juice. If you are at an international restaurant and are unsure of what a meal description actually means — ask what's in it. If you think a dish may be salty ask for it to be prepared without salt.

SMORGASBORDS

These are a good choice because you have more control over the quantity and type of food that goes on your plate.

BISTROS

Choose fish or a small fillet steak rather than an enormous slab of rump (or share one between two people). Kebabs with meat and vegetables or fruit are a good choice. At the salad bar eat plenty of the low fat selections but be sparing with those laden with dressings.

ASIAN FOODS

Preferably have steamed dim sims rather than deep fried, chow mein rather than deep fried honey king prawns, lychees rather than fried ice cream and so on. Choose restaurants that don't use MSG and ask them to avoid salt in the preparation of your meal.

DESSERT

Fresh fruits such as strawberries or fruit salads, frozen fruit desserts, sorbet, gelatin desserts. Avoid the fatty ones — ice cream, cream, pies, pastries, chocolate, etc.

BREADS

Breads are a good choice when you are out because they are filling. Go easy on garlic and herb breads because of their added fat.

DRINKS

Don't forget that alcohol is an appetite stimulant. Pre-dinner drinks not only add calories to the outing, they make you hungrier and you tend to eat more. Stick to Harry's Rule of Twos. Preferably have low calorie drinks and order a jug of iced water.

Bon Appetit

Recipe Alternatives

SPAGHETTI BOLOGNAISE

Serves 6

- **Less fat.** Buy lean meat, buy less meat, remove fat in preparation and/or cooking; oil is not used in cooking; small serving of sauce.
- **Less salt.** None added during cooking; buy 'no added salt' products; adding extra garlic and herbs boosts flavour in the absence of salt.
- **More fibre.** Substitute beans for a portion of the meat (the sceptics in your family won't even know if you mash or blend them); more vegetables; use wholemeal pasta if you like it.

And it still tastes great!

Whoo up! What about the Parmesan cheese? A light dusting is fine. Parmesan cheese is high in fat and salt but because it has a strong flavour you only need a small amount to appreciate the flavour.

NOT SO HEALTHY	HEALTHY
750 g of mince steak *1 large onion* *½ capsicum* *1 can of tomatoes* *1 clove of garlic* *2 tablespoons tomato paste* *2 tablespoons olive oil* *½ teaspoon salt* *½ cup red wine* *basil, oregano* *200 g spaghetti* *2 teaspoons salt* Brown mince in half the oil and set aside. Sauté finely chopped onion, capsicum and crushed garlic in remaining oil. Add meat, tomatoes, tomato paste, salt and herbs. Simmer for one hour. Add wine ten minutes before serving. Cook spaghetti in boiling water and salt. Serve a large helping of sauce on a small bed of spaghetti. Serve with a bottle or two of full bodied red wine. 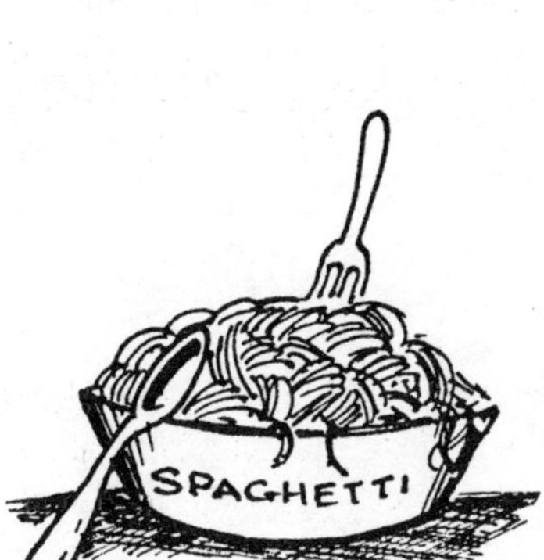 	***400 g lean mince steak*** ***340 g can of red kidney beans, rinsed and roughly mashed or blended*** ***2 large onions*** ***1 capsicum*** ***2 cloves garlic*** ***1 can tomatoes (no added salt)*** ***2 tablespoons tomato paste (no added salt)*** ***1 teaspoon oregano*** ***1 teaspoon basil*** ***1 tablespoon parsley*** ***1 tablespoon chives*** ***½ cup of red wine (optional)*** ***250 g wholemeal spaghetti*** **Cook meat early in ¼ cup of water. Skim off fat by tilting the pan and spooning away half the water. Sauté finely chopped onion and capsicum and crushed garlic in a little water (best in a non-stick fry pan). Add meat, beans, tomatoes, tomato paste and herbs. Simmer for one hour (the longer the better). Boil spaghetti in water.** **Serve a medium helping of sauce on a large bed of spaghetti.** **Cooking with wine is OK as most of the alcohol is evaporated.** **A full bodied red wine would be a fine accompaniment *but* don't forget Harry's Rule of Twos.**

MEAT AND THREE (or four or five) VEGES

Meat and three veges is probably the most common meal served in Australia. If this is your style of meal you may not enjoy cooking totally different meals for the sake of your health and you don't have to. Yes, you will have to reduce the amount of fat in the meal but you don't have to switch to a fare that may not suit you.

NOT SO HEALTHY	HEALTHY
150 to 450 g of steak, sausages, chops, lamb or pork.	***90 to 150 g of lean meat — steak, veal, chops without fat, lamb or pork.***
The meat is cooked in the fry pan and often oil or fat is added.	**Cut fat from meat before cooking and grill on a rack.**
The meat is usually the most abundant food on the plate and fat is eaten.	**Meat is not the most abundant food on the plate. It is important to put more of something else on the plate to make up the difference or you will leave the table still hungry. Don't simply add more of the same vegetables the meal will become boring. Add one or two new varieties. Have some bread with the meal.**
Two types of vegetables boiled in salty water and chips which are deep fried in oil.	**Four or five different veges steamed, dry baked or microwaved.**
Oven fries are cooked in the oven but have fat added in their processing.	

No fuss and much the same!

ROAST CHICKEN

Serves 6

It's not so long ago that chicken was a real treat but today most families eat it at least once a week. Chicken is fine as long as you prepare it in a healthy fashion, which means removing the skin and fat before you cook it and not using oil in the cooking process. For chicken casseroles, curries and soups your Good Eating Guidelines make very little difference to the taste or appearance of the meal. Unfortunately it's not the same for the traditional roast chicken. Try the healthy alternative below but if you are not satisfied try other ways of cooking chicken.

NOT SO HEALTHY	HEALTHY
1 chicken *oil* *vegetables* Chicken is placed in the bottom of a baking pan with oil and roasted in a hot oven. Baste regularly with pan juices. Vegetables are added early in the cooking and roasted in the bottom of the baking pan. A gravy is made from the pan juices.	***1 chicken with skin and visible fat removed*** ***vegetables*** **Add water to the baking dish and place the chicken on a rack above the water. Baste regularly with pan juices. You may add herbs to the water to add flavour.** **When cooked remove the chicken and reduce the pan juices, spoon off any fat and then make a gravy.** **Cook the vegetables separately by either dry baking, steaming or microwaving.**

Italian Chicken

Serves 4

8 small chicken pieces, skinned and visible fat removed

2 onions sliced in rings

2 cloves of garlic

3 tomatoes, chopped

2 cups mushrooms, sliced

1 tablespoon of tomato paste

$^1/_3$ cup water

$^1/_3$ teaspoon basil and oregano

cornflour

optional —
2 tablespoons of brandy

Place chicken, onion and garlic in a pan with a little water. Cook for 15 minutes on a medium heat. Add other ingredients except brandy and cook gently for a further 30 to 40 minutes.

Thicken with cornflour, if necessary.

Add brandy just before cooking is finished.

Serve with rice, pasta or vegetables and a green side salad.

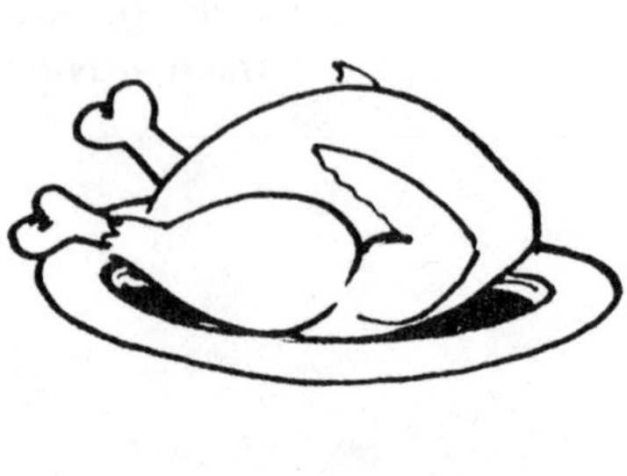

Whole Chicken in Vegetable Sauce Serves 6

1 chicken, skinned and visible fat removed

1 can 'no added salt' tomatoes or 3 fresh tomatoes, chopped

1 cup grated zucchini

1 large onion, finely chopped

1 tablespoon 'no added salt' tomato paste

herbs as you like — suggest garlic, basil and oregano

cornflour

Place chicken in the bottom of a baking dish with a little water and roast for 15 minutes. Cover with other ingredients and roast until the chicken is cooked. Regularly spoon sauce over the chicken. Add water if necessary.

Before serving, remove the chicken and thicken the sauce with cornflour.

Serve with noodles (try some of the fancy styles such as vegeroni and soyaroni), with brown rice or more vegetables.

But what about thickening sauces if you are on a diet? You won't get many calories from one spoon of humble cornflour shared among six people.

Annette's Tropical Chicken Serves 4

8 small chicken pieces, skinned and visible fat removed

2 onions, sliced in rings

1 small can unsweetened pineapple pieces, use half the juice

2 sticks celery, chopped

1 red capsicum, sliced in thin strips

2 carrots, cut in thin sticks

1 cup mushrooms, sliced

1 dessertspoon of cornflour

optional — 1 dessertspoon reduced salt soya sauce

Place chicken and onion in a pan with a little water. Cover and cook for 15 minutes on a medium heat. Add other ingredients and cook gently for a further 30 to 40 minutes. Thicken with cornflour.

Serve with rice, pasta or vegetables.

Serve a side dish of fresh pineapple, rockmelon, grapes and passionfruit halves. Spectacular but simple.

It tastes magnificent. I have to say that because Annette is my wife.

Fish with Tomatoes

Serves 4

700 g white fish fillets (for example gem, ling, perch)

2 onions, sliced in rings

2 large tomatoes, thinly sliced

1 tablespoon 'no added salt' tomato paste

1 teaspoon tarragon

Sauté onion in a little water. Add fish, tomatoes and tomato paste. Cover and cook for 15 minutes or until fish flakes easily. Add tarragon five minutes before the fish is cooked. Serve with rice or spiral noodles and crusty bread.

Fillets in Foil

Serves 4

4 x 180 g white fish fillets

8 king prawns (cooked or green)

8 Tasmanian scallops

2 lemons

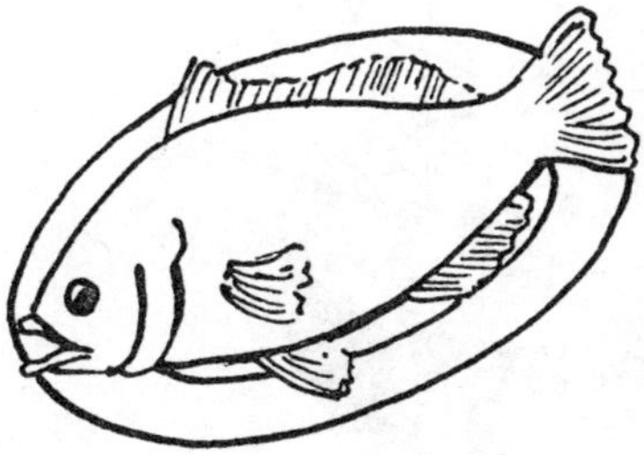

Place each piece of fish on a square of sturdy aluminium foil. On the fish place two prawns and two scallops. Fold the sides of the foil around the fish and squeeze the juice of half a lemon into each. Crush the edges of the foil together above the fish to form a bag. Place in a baking dish and cook in an oven or cook directly on the barbecue plate. Take care not to puncture the foil bag. Fish is cooked when it flakes easily.

Serve by opening the foil bags and eat the fish from them. Use a spoon to help yourself to the delightful soup the fish is cooked in.

This is a very simple yet quite entertaining meal. It's not expensive as you are only buying a few prawns and scallops. Don't worry about the cholesterol in the prawns, this small quantity won't make any difference.

Minestrone

Serves 8

3 cups cooked dried beans (red kidney, haricot, black eye, chick peas or you may prefer a mixture)

4 thin slices of hot salami, finely chopped

2 large onions, chopped

3 cloves garlic, chopped

3 cups celery, chopped

3 carrots, diced

1½ cups shredded cabbage

2 zucchini, chopped

6 cups chicken stock or water

2 x 425 g cans 'no added salt' tomatoes

3 tablespoons 'no added salt' tomato paste

3 tablespoons chopped fresh parsley

1 teaspoon mixed herbs

½ cup brown rice

Put all ingredients except beans in a large pot and bring to the boil. Reduce heat and simmer for one hour before adding beans and serving.

Note: Cooking Dried Beans

Place beans in a saucepan and cover well with water. Bring to the boil for two minutes. Remove from heat and let stand overnight. Next day, heat and cook for one to three hours until tender. Cooking time varies between varieties, black eye beans may only need an hour whereas soya beans may require three hours.

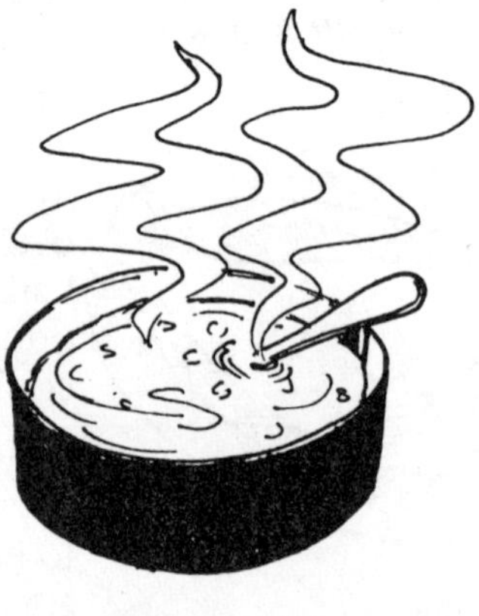

But salami is high in fat! True, but this is a good example of how you can take advantage of strong tasting foods that are not so healthy. You only need a very small amount so the total amount of fat in this meal is still very small.

Veal and Chick Pea Casserole

Serves 6

800 g of veal (beef or lamb may substitute)

2 cups cooked chick peas

1 large onion, chopped

3 cloves garlic, crushed

2 tablespoons plain wholemeal flour

1 x 425 g can 'no added salt' tomatoes

1 cup 'no added salt' tomato juice

juice of 1 lemon

8 eschallots

3 dessertspoons chopped fresh parsley or chives

black pepper to taste

½ cup low fat yoghurt

1 tablespoon chopped fresh parsley

Trim fat from meat and cut into 2 cm cubes. In a non stick pan sauté onions and garlic in water. Coat meat with flour then add to pan and stir for two minutes. Place all ingredients except yoghurt and parsley into a casserole. Bake in moderate oven for one and a half hours.

Stir in yoghurt and sprinkle with parsley or chives before serving.

Serve with jacket potatoes and steamed vegetables.

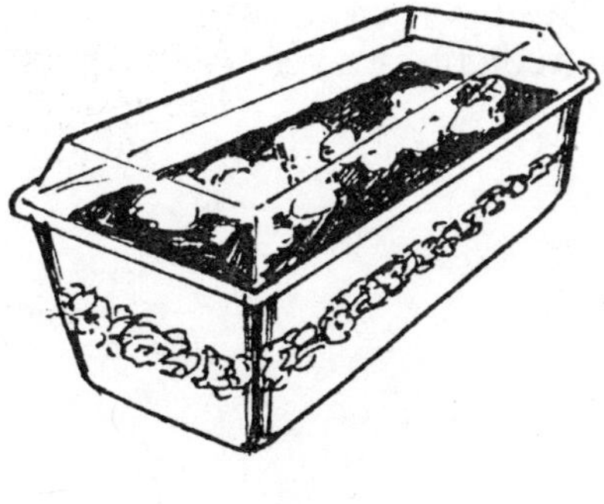

Curried Vegetables

Serves 4

2 cups of chicken stock

1 onion, finely chopped

1 clove of garlic, crushed

1 teaspoon turmeric

½ teaspoon chilli powder

1 teaspoon coriander

2 large tomatoes, chopped

1 tablespoon dried coconut

1 cup each of carrot strips, green beans in 2 cm lengths, red capsicum strips, broccoli and cauliflower rosettes, green peas, zucchini slices, chopped apple and button mushrooms

Bring stock to the boil, add onion, tomato and spices and simmer for five minutes. Add vegetables and coconut then simmer until vegetables are tender but not overcooked.

Serve with rice and a tossed salad.

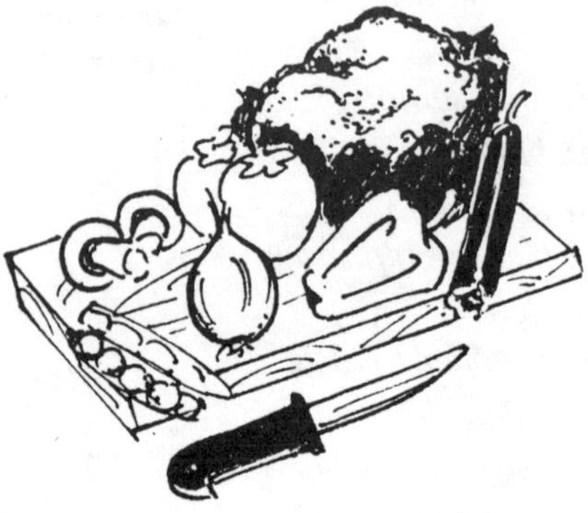

But coconut is high in saturated fat! This is true and you should use coconut sparingly. It's reasonable to include it in a meal such as this because you are using a relatively small quantity and the other ingredients are very low in fat.

Homemade Pizza

Serves 4

Base

1 large Lebanese bread

Topping

2 tablespoons of 'no added salt' tomato paste (better still left over bolognaise sauce)

½ cup cottage or ricotta cheese

1 onion, finely sliced in rings

½ capsicum, cut in thin strips

½ cup sliced mushrooms

½ teaspoon oregano and basil

1 tablespoon parmesan cheese

Spread bread with tomato paste or bolognaise sauce. Cover with cottage or ricotta cheese. Arrange other vegetables on top and sprinkle with herbs and parmesan cheese. Cook in a hot oven for 15 minutes.

Serve with plenty of tossed salad.

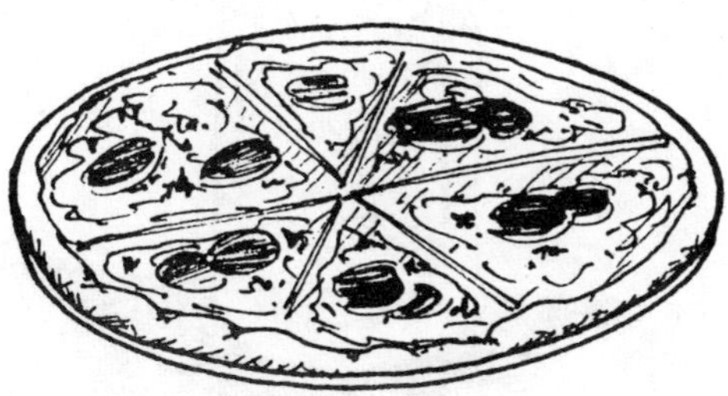

Mayonnaise

Makes 1½ cups

½ cup low fat natural yoghurt

½ cup low fat ricotta (or cottage) cheese

3 tablespoons vinegar

1 tablespoon lemon juice

¼ teaspoon garlic powder

¼ teaspoon mustard powder

Put all the ingredients in a blender and blend.

Variations

- Chive mayonnaise — fold in half cup of chives after blending. You may or may not want to include the mustard powder.
- Seafood dressing — substitute tomato sauce for the mustard powder.

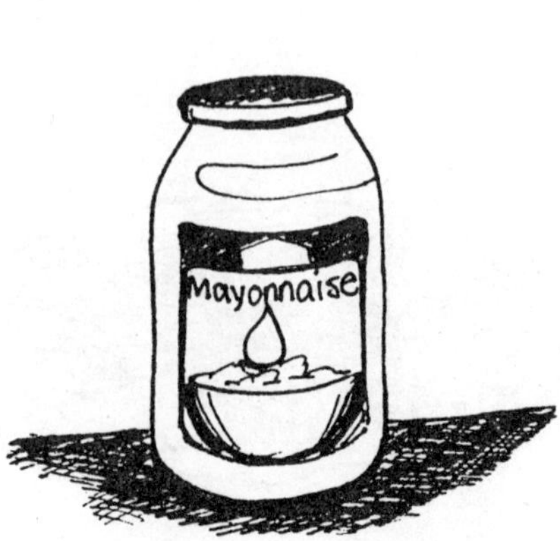

Coleslaw

Serves 4

2 cups cabbage, shredded

½ cup celery, chopped

½ cup carrot, grated

½ cup pineapple, chopped

½ cup red capsicum, chopped

¼ cup walnuts, chopped

½ cup apple, chopped

½ cup Mayonnaise (see recipe)

Combine all ingredients and fold the mayonnaise into the mixture.

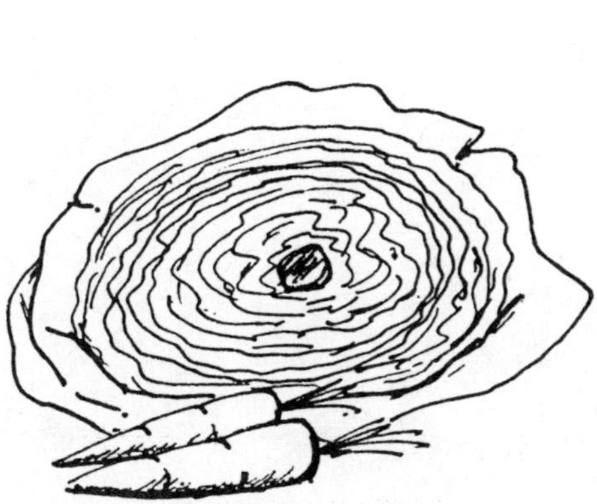

Party Dips

Sour Cream Substitute Blend low fat ricotta with skim milk or low fat natural yoghurt. Adjust quantity of milk or yoghurt to determine thickness of the dip.

Variations

- Chilli dip — blend in chilli powder to your taste or fold in hot taco sauce.
- French onion dip — blend in a packet of reduced salt French onion soup.
- Corn dip — after blending, fold in some corn relish.
- Crab meat dip — after blending, fold in a can of well-drained crab meat. Harry has been known to add a dessertspoon of brandy to this one.

When using foods like crab meat, corn relish, taco sauce and so on you need not worry too much about the salt content. These products usually don't account for a large percentage of people's total salt intake. Certainly if there is a 'no added salt' or 'reduced salt' alternative available use it.

Bran Muffins

Makes approximately 8

1½ cups wholemeal self raising flour

1 cup low fat, sugar free, flavoured yoghurt

¼ cup unprocessed wheat or oat bran

¼ cup skim milk powder

1 egg

1 cup sultanas

½ cup unsweetened grape juice

Preheat oven. Combine all the ingredients. Place spoonfuls into non-stick muffin tins.

Bake in a moderate oven for 15 to 20 minutes until brown.

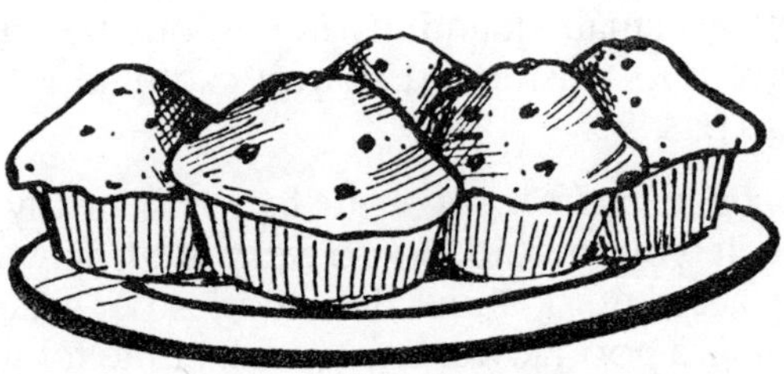

Dorothy's Date Loaf (A fibre feast) Serves 4

2 cups All Bran

2 cups skim milk

2 dessertspoons golden syrup

2 cups wholemeal self raising flour (use white flour if you feel the loaves are too heavy)

1½ cups chopped dates (you can use any dried fruit you prefer)

1 cup chopped walnuts or pecan nuts

5 x 440 g cans baked beans

You only need the baked beans for the cans, which means that you have to plan 5 high fibre meals in advance — what a bonus. Alternatively, use round loaf tins.

Soak All Bran in milk and golden syrup for at least 3 hours (preferably overnight).

Mix in flour, nuts and dates. Two thirds fill each can. Cover with aluminium foil and secure with string. Stand cans in a covered saucepan with water one third the depth of the cans. Bring water to the boil then simmer for 1½ hours. Remove from heat and stand cans in cold water for 15 minutes. Run knife around the edge of the cans and the loaves will turn out easily.

Serve with custard made from skim milk for dessert or use in moderation instead of biscuits and cake.

But nuts have a high oil content! Nuts are a nutritious food but they do contain oil so they should be used sparingly. In a recipe such as this you are getting very little oil per serve. Eating nuts in small quantities is OK but be careful not to have a jar of nuts positioned so you can grab a handful each time you go past it.

Golden syrup is high in sugar! In fact it is nearly all sugar so if you use it you should do so very sparingly. In this case it will only account for about five calories per slice. Apple juice concentrate is a good lower energy substitute for golden syrup, honey and sugar in cooking. You may try it in this recipe. Alternatively artificial sweeteners may be used.

This recipe comes with rules:

Rule 1 Give two of the loaves away to friends. It cuts down on calories and it puts a smile on someone else's face.

Rule 2 Throw away the empty baked bean cans after you have made the loaves. This increases your fibre intake because you have to eat another five cans of baked beans before you can make another batch of loaves.

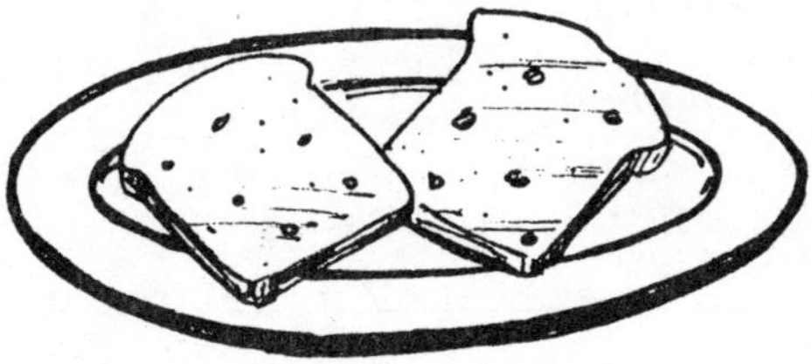

Strawberry Cream

Makes 1½ cups

1 cup low-fat ricotta cheese

½ cup skim milk (adjust quantity to determine thickness)

½ cup fresh strawberries

Place all ingredients into a blender and blend.

Serve with fresh, stewed or canned fruit or wherever else you would have previously used sweet cream.

Variations:

- Apricots, peaches, mangos, plums, bananas may be substituted for the strawberries.
- Fold in the pulp of two passionfruits.
- Add one teaspoon of vanilla essence.

Vanilla Rice Pudding

Serves 4

1½ cups cooked brown rice

1 apple, sliced thinly

1/3 cup condensed skim milk

1 egg, beaten

½ teaspoon vanilla essence

1/3 teaspoon cinnamon

Mix rice, egg, condensed milk and vanilla and place in a flat ovenproof dish. Cover with thin slices of apple and dust with cinnamon. Bake uncovered for 30 minutes.

Serve with cream substitute, stewed fruit or fruit canned in natural juice.

Porridge

Rolled oats is a very healthy and filling breakfast but it may lose some of its appeal if you don't use salt in the cooking and don't pile on some brown sugar. Here are some healthy suggestions that will make porridge popular again.

- Cook the oats in skim milk rather than water.
- Mix in low fat flavoured yoghurt.
- Cook in some grated apple, chopped pear, grapes, flaked almonds, sultanas or any other dried fruits.

Quick and Easy Muesli

500 g rolled oats

375 g oat or wheat bran

1½ cups currants

1½ cups dried fruit medley, chopped

1 cup unsalted mixed nuts, chopped

1 cup dates, chopped

Mix all ingredients together and store in sealed containers.

Enjoyable, healthy and very easy to make.

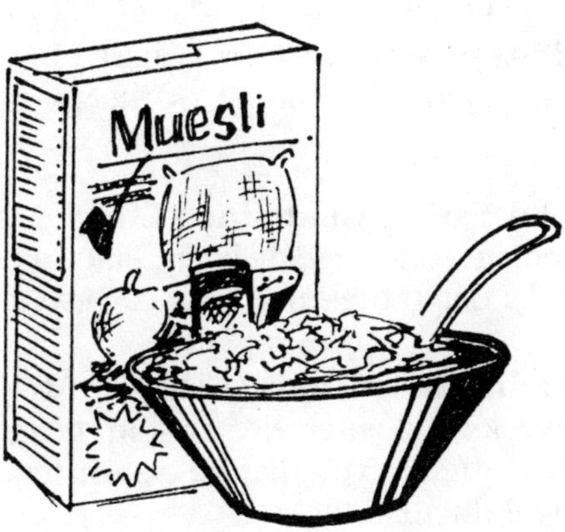

Record Section

The Charts

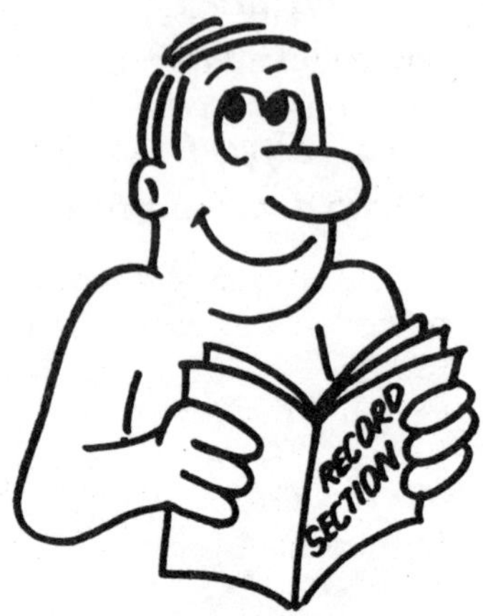

You will make regular entries in this Record Section for the following 20 weeks. It is not a novelty add-on to the book but rather it is the centrepiece of the program. The reasons for making entries in your Record Section are to keep track of your progress through the program and, most importantly, to provide you with daily prompts or behavioural cues. Each time you make an entry in the Record Section you are subconsciously telling yourself — 'Hey! I am doing something to improve my health.' The charts do take up a considerable portion of the book; don't be put off. They are very simple to use and take up *very little* of your *time*.

Self Assessment Chart (Chart 1). You will make one set of entries at the beginning of the program and another at Week 20.

Good Eating Guidelines Check List (Chart 2). You will make entries on a weekly basis. Place a note in your diary or on the calendar at the same time each week as a reminder.

Weight Loss Graph (Chart 3). Weigh yourself once every two weeks and enter the result in the graph. Don't weigh yourself more often as you may be disheartened by your body's natural weight fluctuations.

Physical Activity Diary (Chart 4). Each day enter any fitness activity you do and the time you spend doing it.

Quit Check List (Chart 5). If you are a smoker enter the number of cigarettes you smoke each day.

Harry's Rule of Twos (Chart 6). Enter the number of alcoholic drinks you have each day.

The Way I Think Check List (Chart 7). Tick each day you read through your list of 'affirmations' (page 83).

Time Outs Check List (Chart 8). Enter the number of time outs you take each day.

Average Blood Pressure Graphs (Chart 10). You will make entries into these graphs each time you have accumulated five recordings in your **Blood Pressure Tables** (Chart 9).

Timetable (Chart 11). You will make several entries in the first few weeks of the program.

Date Chart (Chart 12). You will make entries once only at the beginning of the program. The Date Chart gives the program a time frame. Week 1, etc. become specific dates for your personal program.

YEARLY

This program really is a long term project. Some of the charts have been designed so you can update them once each year for the next ten years. Right now go to your calendar or diary and enter the following reminder note at the beginning of next December — Update my *Better Blood Pressure* charts. When December arrives dust this book off and update your progress. Weigh yourself, take your blood pressure, check your Good Eating Guidelines and so on. Place the entries under Year Number 1. When you have done this place an entry in your new calendar or diary to remind you to repeat the process next year.

Self Assessment

To successfully complete any journey you need to know:

- where you are — **Before**
- where you want to be — **Ideal**
- where you end up — **After**

Before is your current physical condition. By reviewing your current physical condition you will get an insight into the reasons behind your blood pressure situation.

Ideal is the physical condition that will provide you with the best possible chance of achieving 'your aim'.

After is your physical condition at Week 20 (or at any time in the future). You are aiming to make *after* match *ideal*.

This chapter will help you to establish your *before, ideal* and *after* for:

- systolic and diastolic blood pressure
- body weight
- physical activity
- alcohol consumption
- cigarette consumption
- salt consumption
- stress management ability

Work through this Self Assessment filling in your Self Assessment Chart on page 132 as you go. Have your Self Assessment Chart completed, as best you can, before continuing with the program.

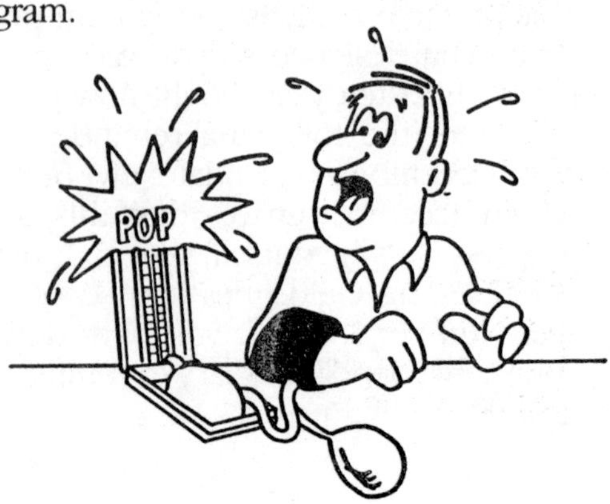

BLOOD PRESSURE

Before. Enter your average systolic and average diastolic pressures in the *before* column of your Self Assessment Chart. To calculate average pressure you will need five or more blood pressure recordings, recorded on separate days. Use the table below to help you make the calculation.

Average blood pressure equals the total of recordings divided by the number of recordings. For example if your five recordings were:

150/100 140/95 140/100 170/105 150/95

Average Systolic
BP = 150 + 140 + 140 + 170 + 150 = 750 ÷5 = 150

Average Diastolic
BP = 100 + 95 + 100 + 105 + 95 = 495 ÷5 = 99

Write your blood pressure recordings here:

Systolic =____+____+____+____+____=____÷5=____

Diastolic=____+____+____+____+____=____÷5=____

If you have more than five recordings use them but remember to divide by the number of recordings. The more recordings you have the better.

Ideal. Your Self Assessment Chart has *ideal* blood pressures printed. We will consider the *ideal* range for systolic pressure to be 100 to 135 and for diastolic pressure to be 60 to 85. **Please Note:** If you are taking blood pressure medication you may already be within these limits. You may consider your *ideal* situation to be within these limits without the need for any or as much medication. If this is the case you should share your intentions with your doctor and only make decisions about medication levels with his or her consultation.

After. After Week 20 select five or preferably more blood pressure recordings and calculate average systolic and diastolic blood pressures. Enter the results in the *after* column of your Self Assessment Chart.

BODY WEIGHT

Before. Weigh yourself on scales that are reasonably accurate and that you will have access to during the program. When weighing yourself wear only light clothing and no shoes. Enter your weight in the *before* column of your Self Assessment Chart.

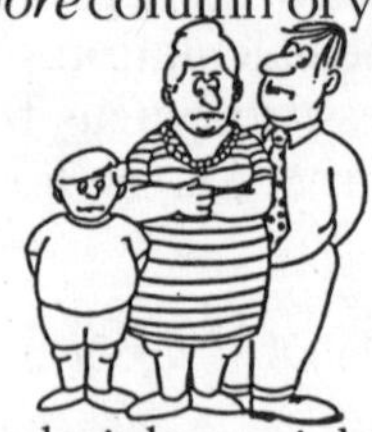

Ideal. The following height weight table will assist you to choose your ideal body weight.

If you are above your ideal range you will need to lose some weight. If you are in the ideal range but feel you are still a little overweight you are probably right. The 'grab test' may help you decide. If you grab your waist and there is a handful to grab you may still need to lose some weight. If this is the case you should choose a new ideal range that you believe is correct for you, perhaps 2 kg either side of the lower number indicated by the table. Don't be unrealistic by choosing an ideal weight range that is out of reach.

When selecting your frame size it is wise to confirm your selection with someone else.

After. After Week 20 weigh yourself and enter your weight in the after column of your Self Assessment Chart.

Before continuing enter your weight in your Weight Loss Graph. You will notice there is no weight scale — you have to write the scale to suit your needs. On the top left corner of the graph write in a weight 1 kg heavier than you are now. Then count backwards down the column, writing in the numbers as you go until you reach the lower number of your ideal weight range. If you are more than 12 kg heavier than the top number of your ideal weight range allow one space on the graph to equal 2 kg. Highlight your ideal weight range across the graph.

Place a mark in the Week 1 column at your present weight.

HEIGHT WEIGHT TABLE							
WOMEN				MEN			
HEIGHT (No Shoes)	SMALL FRAME	MEDIUM FRAME	LARGE FRAME	HEIGHT (No Shoes)	SMALL FRAME	MEDIUM FRAME	LARGE FRAME
cm	kg	kg	kg	cm	kg	kg	kg
143	42-44	44-49	47-54	155	51-54	54-59	57-64
145	43-46	45-50	48-55	158	52-56	55-60	59-65
148	44-48	46-51	49-57	160	53-57	56-62	60-67
150	45-49	47-53	51-58	163	55-58	58-63	61-69
153	46-50	49-54	52-59	165	56-60	59-65	63-71
155	48-51	50-55	53-61	168	58-62	61-67	64-73
158	49-53	51-57	55-63	170	60-64	63-69	67-75
160	50-54	53-59	57-64	173	62-66	64-71	68-77
163	52-56	54-61	59-66	175	64-68	66-73	70-79
165	54-58	56-63	60-68	178	65-70	68-75	72-81
168	55-59	58-65	62-70	180	67-72	70-77	74-84
170	57-61	60-67	64-72	183	69-74	72-79	76-86
173	59-63	62-69	66-74	185	71-76	74-82	78-88
175	61-65	63-70	68-76	188	73-78	76-84	81-90
178	63-67	65-72	69-79	190	74-79	78-86	83-93

Reproduced from *The Australian Pocket Calorie Counter* Allan Borushek, 1985

PHYSICAL ACTIVITY

The Activity Scorer that follows will help you assess your level of physical activity. This in turn is an indication of your physical fitness. The Activity Scorer is a personal rating system not a scientific fitness measuring device. It is not a valid means of comparing your fitness with other people.

Read through the Activity Scorer and complete the table that follows it.

Use your discretion when working through the Activity Scorer and give yourself fair approximations of the score each particular activity deserves. The scores are for *15 minutes* of the particular activity (except walking which is *20 minutes*). If you do the activity for 30 minutes (walking for 40 minutes), simply double the score. *You may only score up to 60 minutes of an activity per day.* You must have been doing the activity on a regular basis, for at least the *past six weeks* for it to be included.

- **Mild** is a level that you are very comfortable with. You are not breathing very hard and probably not raising a sweat.
- **Brisk** is a level where you feel yourself puffing, you may be raising a sweat. The activity is not so intense that you could not comfortably have a conversation with someone who is doing the activity with you. This is the ideal intensity to exercise safely and gain adequate fitness benefit.
- **Intense** is a level where you are exercising very hard. You are breathing very heavily and probably sweating profusely. You find it difficult to hold a conversation while doing the activity. You should not exercise at this level unless you train to do so. This level is certainly not for people who are seeking to improve a relatively low level of fitness.

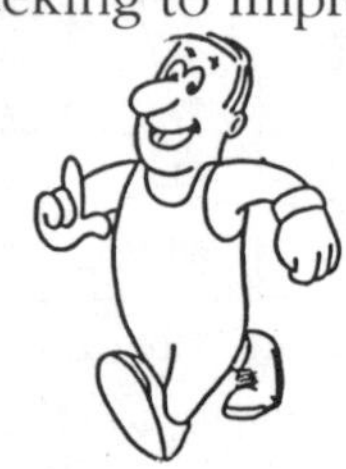

ACTIVITY SCORER

ACTIVITY	INTENSITY	SCORE
walking — (the walk should be continuous for at least 20 minutes)	MILD a leisurely stroll or walking the dog	1
	BRISK walking at a deliberate pace	2
	INTENSE very hard and find it difficult to keep the pace up	3
swimming	MILD easy pace and stopping for rests	1
	BRISK continuous swimming or walking in the water	2
	INTENSE competitive	3

jogging	**BRISK** it is difficult to jog less than a brisk pace **INTENSE** very exhausting	2 3
cycling	**MILD** sight seeing pace. Plenty of free wheeling **BRISK** continuous peddling most of the time **INTENSE** very fast	1 2 3
supervised exercise classes	**MILD** very low impact, stretching type classes **BRISK** you can keep up with the instructor **INTENSE** very exhausted and difficult to keep up	1 2 3
tennis, badminton or table tennis	**MILD** doubles or very easy singles **BRISK** singles or competition doubles **INTENSE** competition singles	1 2 3
football, basketball, hockey, touch footy, indoor cricket	**BRISK** for fun **INTENSE** competitive	2 3
golf	Score three points for every nine holes you play. Twelve points is the maximum you can score from golf in one week	
lawn bowls, ten pin bowling	Score one point per 30 minutes. Six points is the maximum you can score from bowls in one week	
other activities not mentioned	**MILD** **BRISK** **INTENSE**	1 2 3
yoga, tai chi, darts, fishing	All great activities for fun and relaxation but they don't contribute to your cardiovascular fitness	

For example:

ACTIVITY	TIME PER SESSION	SCORE
3 brisk walks	20 min each	6
1 mild walk	60 min	3
1 game of singles tennis	60 min	8
1 brisk swim	30 min	4
	WEEKLY ACTIVITY SCORE	21

Before. Using the following table work out your Weekly Activity Score and enter the result in the before column of your Self Assessment Chart.

ACTIVITY	TIME PER SESSION	SCORE
	WEEKLY ACTIVITY SCORE	

Ideal. Your *ideal* Weekly Activity Score is 20 points or greater.

After. At the end of Week 20 use the table below to work out your Weekly Activity Score and enter the result in the after column of your Self Assessment Chart.

ACTIVITY	TIME PER SESSION	SCORE
	WEEKLY ACTIVITY SCORE	

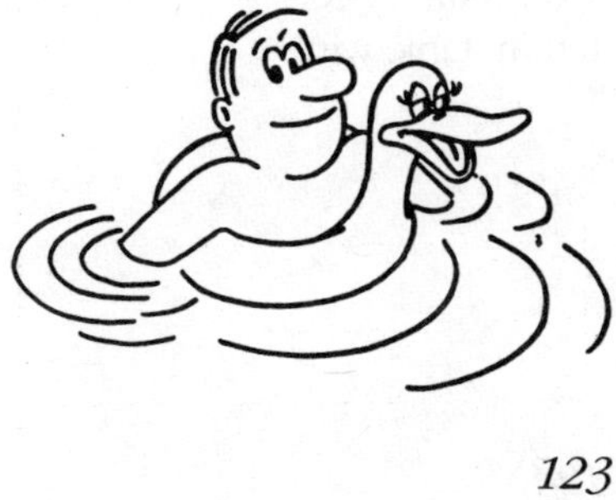

ALCOHOL CONSUMPTION

Before. Estimate your Weekly Alcohol Consumption by completing the following table and enter the result in your Self Assessment Chart. Enter the number of standard drinks you have each day.

SUN	MON	TUE	WED

THUR	FRI	SAT	TOTAL

Ideal. Harry's Rule of Twos (see Not Too Much Grog) is your ideal level of alcohol consumption.

After. At the end of Week 20 use the table below to estimate your Weekly Alcohol Consumption.

SUN	MON	TUE	WED

THUR	FRI	SAT	TOTAL

Standard Drinks

250 ml beer
370 ml light beer
100 ml table wine
60 ml port, sherry, vermouth
30 ml spirits

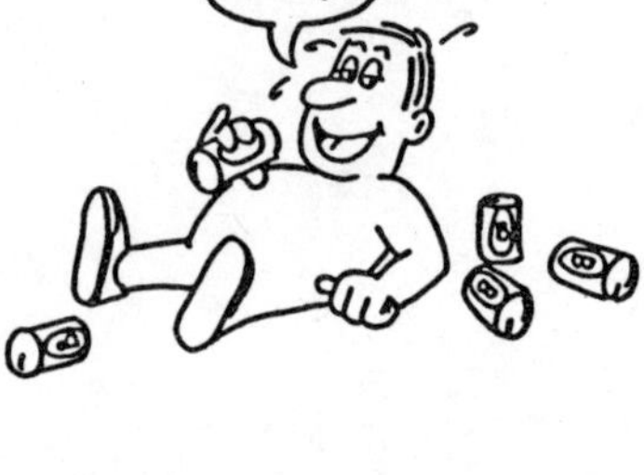

CIGARETTE CONSUMPTION

Before. Estimate your Weekly Cigarette Consumption by completing the following table and enter the result in your Self Assessment Chart.

SUN	MON	TUE	WED

THUR	FRI	SAT	TOTAL

Ideal. Unlike alcohol there is no level of cigarette consumption that is considered safe thus the *ideal* level is nil. You will not be attempting to give up smoking until Week 10. Until then, record the number of cigarettes you smoke each day in the Quit Check List (Chart 5).

After. At the end of Week 20 use the table below to estimate your Weekly Cigarette Consumption. Enter the result in your Self Assessment Chart.

SUN	MON	TUE	WED

THUR	FRI	SAT	TOTAL

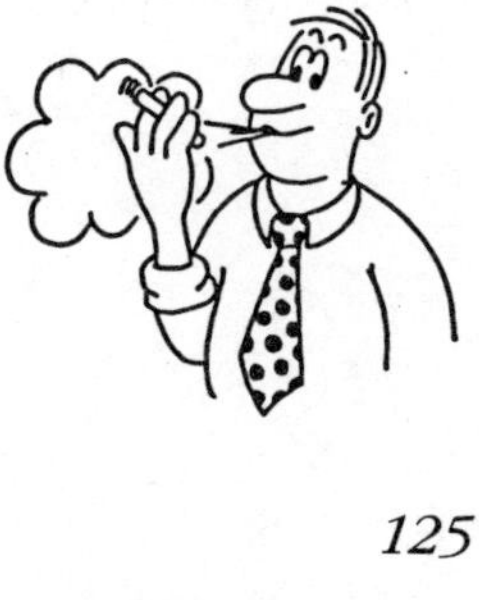

SALT CONSUMPTION

Using the Salt Scorer below, estimate your salt consumption. Circle the number of times you have eaten the following foods in the past three days, not counting today. Fill in the table as accurately as possible, indicating every time you have eaten the food mentioned. Count the occasions not the amounts (for example, three slices of bread score 1, if eaten on one occasion). Score 8 if you have had the food on more than eight occasions. Don't count foods labelled unsalted or no added salt; count a half score if the food is labelled salt reduced.

Before. The Salt Scorer allows you to gain a reasonable indication of your level of salt consumption. Complete it and enter the result in your Self Assessment Chart.

Ideal. A score of 23 or less is ideal.

After. After Week 20 repeat the questionnaire and enter the result in your Self Assessment Chart.

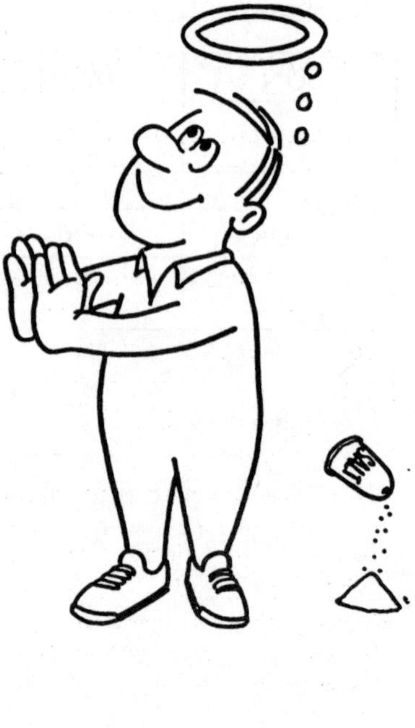

SALT SCORER			
FOOD TYPE	OCCASIONS	Before Score	After Score
food with salt added in the cooking	0 1 2 3 4 5 6 7 8		
food with salt added at table	0 1 2 3 4 5 6 7 8		
cured meats such as ham, bacon, sausages or luncheon meats	0 1 2 3 4 5 6 7 8		
corned/canned meats, salami, meat paste	0 1 2 3 4 5 6 7 8		
pies, pasties or sausage rolls	0 1 2 3 4 5 6 7 8		
canned or smoked fish or fish pastes	0 1 2 3 4 5 6 7 8		
mature cheese, processed cheese or cheese spread	0 1 2 3 4 5 6 7 8		
yeast or vegetable extracts such as Vegemite, Marmite or Promite	0 1 2 3 4 5 6 7 8		
olives, salted nuts, crackers or potato crisps	0 1 2 3 4 5 6 7 8		
canned vegetables or soups	0 1 2 3 4 5 6 7 8		
packet soups, beef/chicken cubes	0 1 2 3 4 5 6 7 8		
dressings, sauces or pickles	0 1 2 3 4 5 6 7 8		
bread	0 1 2 3 4 5 6 7 8		
breakfast cereals with added salt	0 1 2 3 4 5 6 7 8		
cakes, pastries or biscuits	0 1 2 3 4 5 6 7 8		
butter or margarine	0 1 2 3 4 5 6 7 8		
chocolate or salted confectionery	0 1 2 3 4 5 6 7 8		
any other salty foods not mentioned above	0 1 2 3 4 5 6 7 8		
	TOTAL SCORE		

Adapted, with permission, from *The Medical Journal of Australia Vol. 149,* 15 August, 1988

STRESS

The Stress Rating provides an indication of your ability to manage stress.

Before. Complete the Stress Rating and enter the result in the before column of your Self Assessment Chart. Score '0' if the question is not relevant to you.

STRESS RATING	
Answer each question by circling the number that is most relevant to you. Add up your total score. **0 = rarely, 1 = occasionally, 2 = often, 3 = very often**	
Do you move, walk or eat rapidly?	0 1 2 3
Do you find that you don't sleep well?	0 1 2 3
Do you find yourself being irritable with your partner and/or children?	0 1 2 3
Do you grumble about senior managers, or about those working under you?	0 1 2 3
Do you get strong surges of anger or frustration?	0 1 2 3
Do you feel discontented or dissatisfied with the way your life is going in general?	0 1 2 3
Do you have difficulty working with people you don't like?	0 1 2 3
Do you remember wrongs done to you by others?	0 1 2 3
Do you find it difficult to ask for what you want or need, either at home or work?	0 1 2 3
Do you find it difficult to show affection to your partner and/or children?	0 1 2 3
Do you find it difficult to forget about mistakes you made in the past?	0 1 2 3

Do you find it difficult to praise people (at home or at work) for work well done?	0 1 2 3
Do you have negative feelings about your work or job?	0 1 2 3
Do you find it difficult to listen to another person's point of view?	0 1 2 3
Do you worry about the past and the future rather than enjoying the present?	0 1 2 3
Do you find it difficult to be positive about the problems in your life?	0 1 2 3
Do you enjoy putting other people down?	0 1 2 3
Does criticism really upset you, even when you know it's valid?	0 1 2 3
Do you often feel guilty or angry when you have to say no to someone?	0 1 2 3
Do you feel very uncomfortable about admitting mistakes or errors?	0 1 2 3
Do you tend to see colleagues as competitors rather than as members of the same team?	0 1 2 3
Do you feel very uncomfortable about delegating important jobs to someone else because you don't trust anyone to do as good a job as yourself?	0 1 2 3
Do you feel uncomfortable when you meet people for the first time?	0 1 2 3
Do you feel guilty about doing things just for fun?	0 1 2 3
TOTAL	

Ideal. The ideal score is 16 or less.

After. After Week 20 repeat the Stress Rating and enter the result in your Self Assessment Chart.

MEDICATION

You don't need to read this section if you are not taking any medication to control your blood pressure.

In the *before* column of your Self Assessment Chart write the names and doses of the medications you are currently taking.

The *ideal* column has been replaced by a *comments* column. Note any comments that may result from discussions with your doctor regarding medication.

In the *after* column enter the medications you are taking at Week 20.

OPTIONAL ASSESSMENT

Cholesterol, triglyceride, HDL (a carrier of cholesterol in the blood which has a cardio-protective effect), glucose and uric acid are all substances in your blood. Their levels may be an indication of your risk of developing lifestyle related illnesses such as heart disease and diabetes. A blood test is conducted to determine the levels of these substances. By completing this program you may improve the levels of these substances.

If you have had a blood test conducted recently your doctor may have records of some or all of these tests. Your doctor may consider it worthwhile for you to have these tests conducted.

☐ ***You are now ready to take your next step toward being a 'winner'. Make an appointment to do the chapter 'Weigh Less'. It will take approximately 40 minutes.***

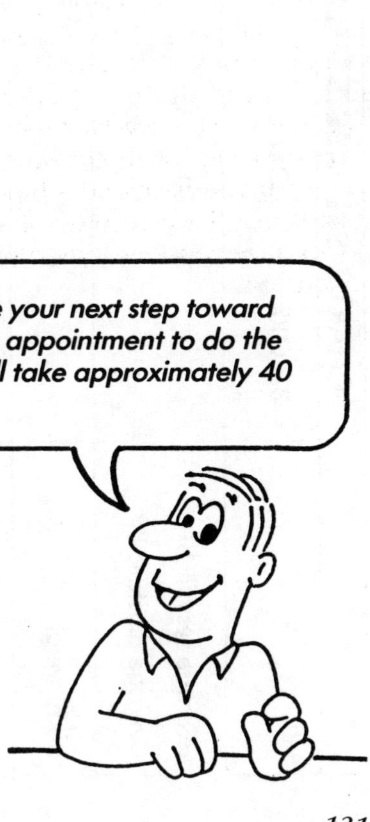

CHART 1: **SELF ASSESSMENT CHART**

	BEFORE	IDEAL	AFTER	YEAR NUMBER									
				1	2	3	4	5	6	7	8	9	10
average systolic BP average diastolic BP		100 — 135 60 — 85											
body weight		to											
weekly activity score		20 or greater											
alcohol consumption		Rule of Twos											
cigarette consumption		nil											
salt consumption		23 or less											
stress rating		16 or less											

MEDICATION		
BEFORE	DOCTORS COMMENTS	AFTER

OPTIONAL ASSESSMENT	BEFORE	IDEAL	AFTER	1	2	3	4	5	6	7	8	9	10
cholesterol		3.0 to 5.5											
triglyceride		0.7 to 2.0											
HDL		0.8 to 2.0											
blood glucose		3.3 to 6.0											
uric acid		0.13 to 0.53											

Normal pathology ranges as per Sydney Diagnostic Services, 1990

CHART 2: **GOOD EATING GUIDELINES CHECK LIST**

Once each week read through the guidelines and tick the ones you are conforming to. Place a cross beside those that you are not conforming to. Don't worry about the crosses, simply work on those guidelines next week.

	Week Number																				Year Number									
	1	2	3	4	5	6	7	8	9	10	11	12	13	14	15	16	17	18	19	20	1	2	3	4	5	6	7	8	9	10
1 DO use wholemeal bread																														
2 DO include a variety of fruits																														
3 DO eat plenty of vegetables																														
4 DO eat a high fibre breakfast																														
5 DO use pasta and rice																														
6 DO try dishes with beans or lentils																														
7 DO eat fruit in preference to juice																														
8 DO buy low fat ingredients																														
9 DO use skim or low fat milk																														
10 LIMIT the amount of all oils you use																														
11 LIMIT cheese																														
12 LIMIT butter and margarine																														
13 AVOID fatty meats																														
14 AVOID cream, sour cream and ice-cream																														
15 AVOID eating biscuits and cakes																														

	Week Number																				Year Number									
	1	2	3	4	5	6	7	8	9	10	11	12	13	14	15	16	17	18	19	20	1	2	3	4	5	6	7	8	9	10
16 AVOID fatty snack foods																														
17 AVOID fatty take-aways																														
18 DO trim meat BEFORE cooking																														
19 DO skin chicken BEFORE cooking																														
20 DO grill or roast rather than frying																														
21 DO allow soups to cool and remove fat																														
22 LIMIT fats and oils when preparing food																														
23 LIMIT amount of meat and chicken																														
24 DO choose 'no added sugar' foods																														
25 AVOID adding sugar to food or drinks																														
26 AVOID high sugar breakfast cereals																														
27 AVOID jams, honey and confectionery																														
28 AVOID soft drinks and cordials																														
29 AVOID adding salt at the table																														
30 AVOID adding salt to cooking																														
31 PREFER 'no added salt' products																														
32 LIMIT salty foods																														

CHART 3: **WEIGHT LOSS GRAPH**

Write down the left hand side of the graph a scale that best suits your weight loss needs. Highlight your ideal weight range. Remember slow, steady and forever.

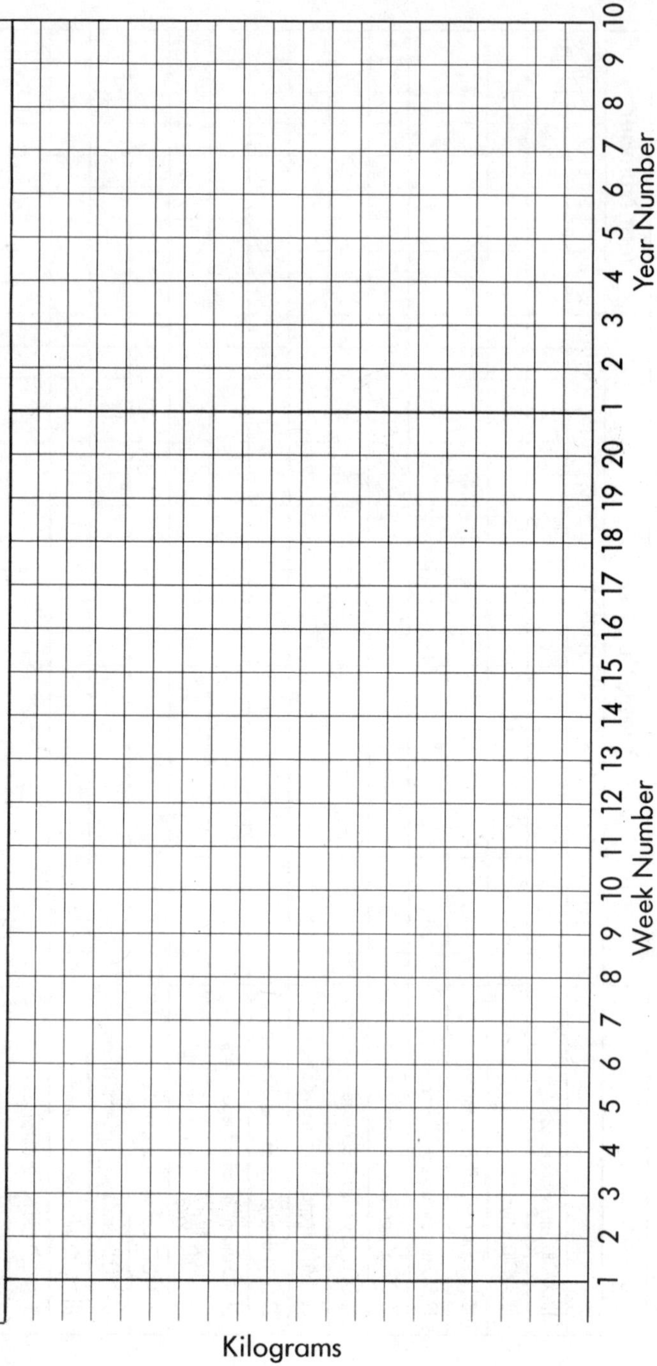

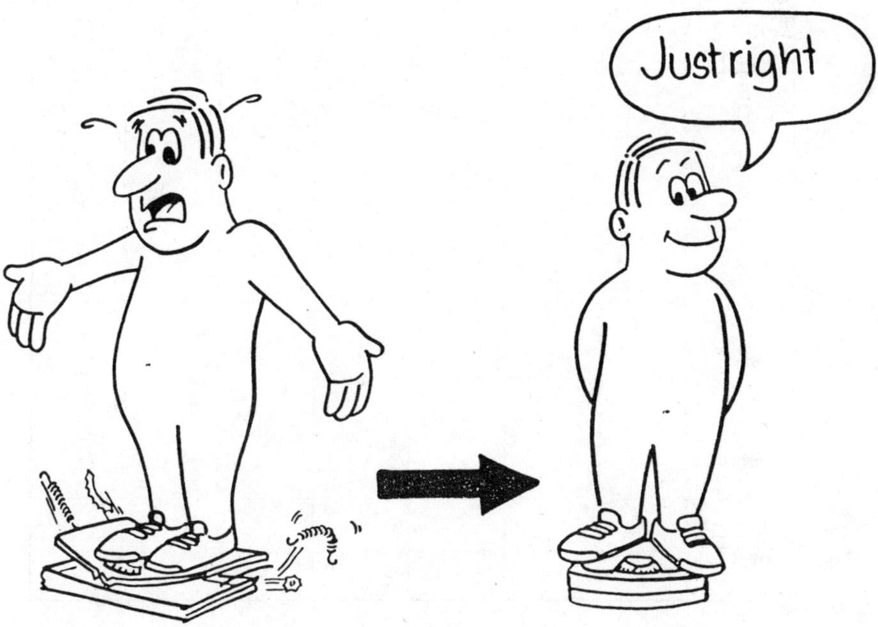
Just right

CHART 4: **MY PHYSICAL ACTIVITY PROGRAM**

The activities I will be doing to improve and then to maintain my fitness levels are:

I intend taking part in these activities to days/week

PHYSICAL ACTIVITY DIARY							
	Sunday	Monday	Tuesday	Wednesday	Thursday	Friday	Saturday
Example	Tennis 60 min	Nil	Walk 40 min	Walk 20 min	Swim 30 min	Nil	Bushwalk 60 min
Week 1							
Week 2							
Week 3							
Week 4							
Week 5							
Week 6							
Week 7							

	Sunday	Monday	Tuesday	Wednesday	Thursday	Friday	Saturday
Week 8							
Week 9							
Week 10							
Week 11							
Week 12							
Week 13							
Week 14							
Week 15							
Week 16							
Week 17							
Week 18							
Week 19							
Week 20							

CHART 5: **QUIT CHECK LIST**

On the ______ / ______ / ______ I begin my new life as a healthy, happy and confident non-smoker.

	Number of cigarettes smoked							
	Sun	Mon	Tue	Wed	Thur	Fri	Sat	Total
Week 1								
Week 2								
Week 3								
Week 4								
Week 5								
Week 6								
Week 7								
Week 8								
Week 9								
I am a healthy, happy and confident non-smoker.								
Week 10								
Week 11								
Week 12								
Week 13								
Week 14								
Week 15								
Week 16								
Week 17								
Week 18								
Week 19								
Week 20								

CHART 6: **HARRY'S RULE of TWOs**

	Number of alcoholic drinks consumed							
	Sun	Mon	Tue	Wed	Thur	Fri	Sat	Total
Week 1								
Week 2								
Week 3								
Week 4								
Week 5								
Two a day is plenty								
Week 6								
Week 7								
Week 8								
Week 9								
Week 10								
Two AFDs a week								
Week 11								
Week 12								
Week 13								
Week 14								
Week 15								
Two — Twos is a treat								
Week 16								
Week 17								
Week 18								
Week 19								
Week 20								
Two treats is too many								

CHART 7: **THE WAY I THINK CHECK LIST**

Place a tick below each day you read through your affirmations.

	Sun	Mon	Tue	Wed	Thur	Fri	Sat
Week 1							
Week 2							
Week 3							
Week 4							
Week 5							
Week 6							
Week 7							
Week 8							
Week 9							
Week 10							
Week 11							
Week 12							
Week 13							
Week 14							
Week 15							
Week 16							
Week 17							
Week 18							
Week 19							
Week 20							

CHART 8: **TIME OUTS CHECK LIST**

Enter the number of time outs you have each day.

	Sun	Mon	Tue	Wed	Thur	Fri	Sat
Week 1							
Week 2							
Week 3							
Week 4							
Week 5							
Week 6							
Week 7							
Week 8							
Week 9							
Week 10							
Week 11							
Week 12							
Week 13							
Week 14							
Week 15							
Week 16							
Week 17							
Week 18							
Week 19							
Week 20							

CHART 9: **BLOOD PRESSURE**

Each time you record your blood pressure enter the date and the recording in a table below. When you have filled a table (five recordings) add the scores and enter the result beside "Total". Divide the total by five to calculate the average systolic and diastolic pressures. Enter the result into your blood pressure graphs by placing a point on the graph above the week in which the fifth recording was taken.

Example

Date	Syst	Diast
8/8	145	85
10/8	145	90
11/8	150	95
13/8	150	85
14/8	145	90
Total	735	445
Average	147	89

Date	Syst	Diast
Total		
Average		

Date	Syst	Diast
Total		
Average		

Date	Syst	Diast
Total		
Average		

Date	Syst	Diast
Total		
Average		

Date	Syst	Diast
Total		
Average		

Date	Syst	Diast
Total		
Average		

Date	Syst	Diast
Total		
Average		

Date	Syst	Diast
Total		
Average		

Date	Syst	Diast
Total		
Average		

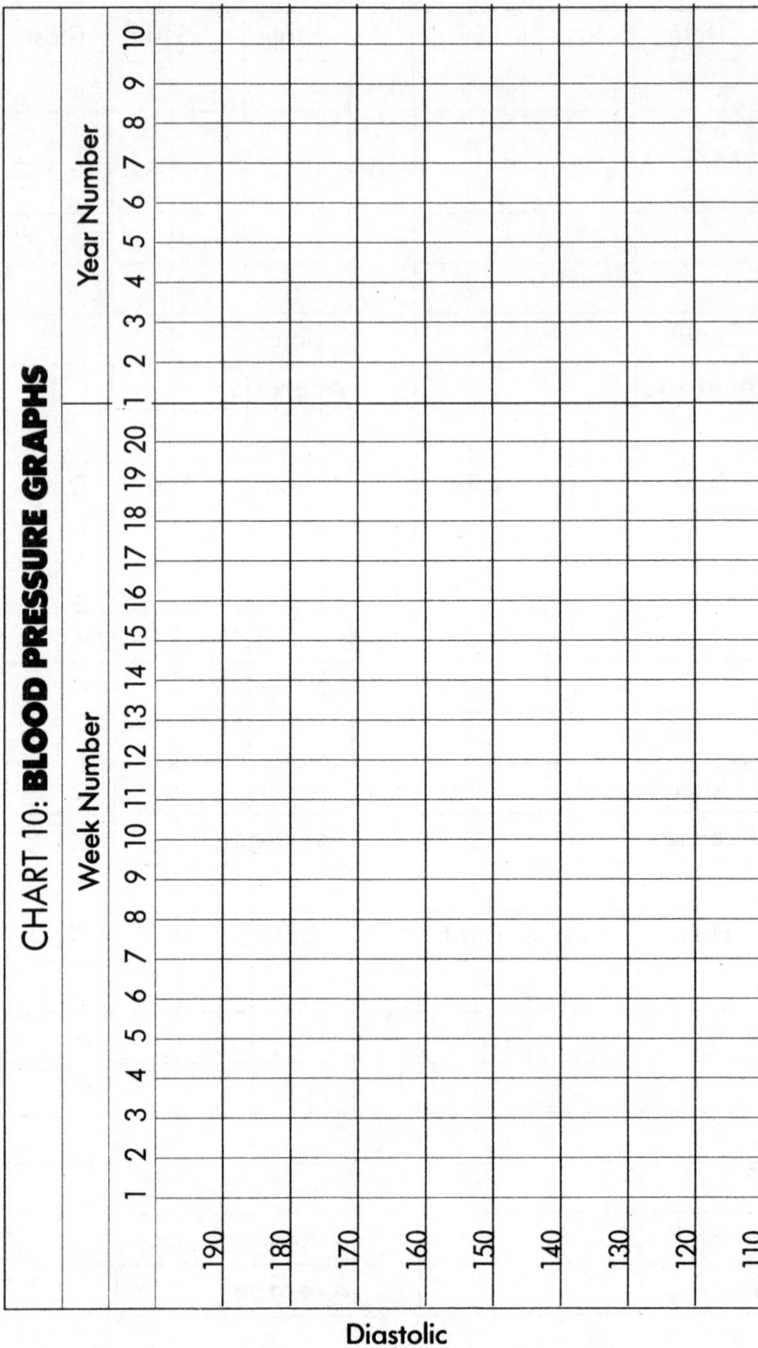
CHART 10: BLOOD PRESSURE GRAPHS
Week Number
1 2 3 4 5 6 7 8 9 10 11 12 13 14 15 16 17 18 19 20
Year Number
1 2 3 4 5 6 7 8 9 10
190
180
170
160
150
140
130
120
110
Diastolic

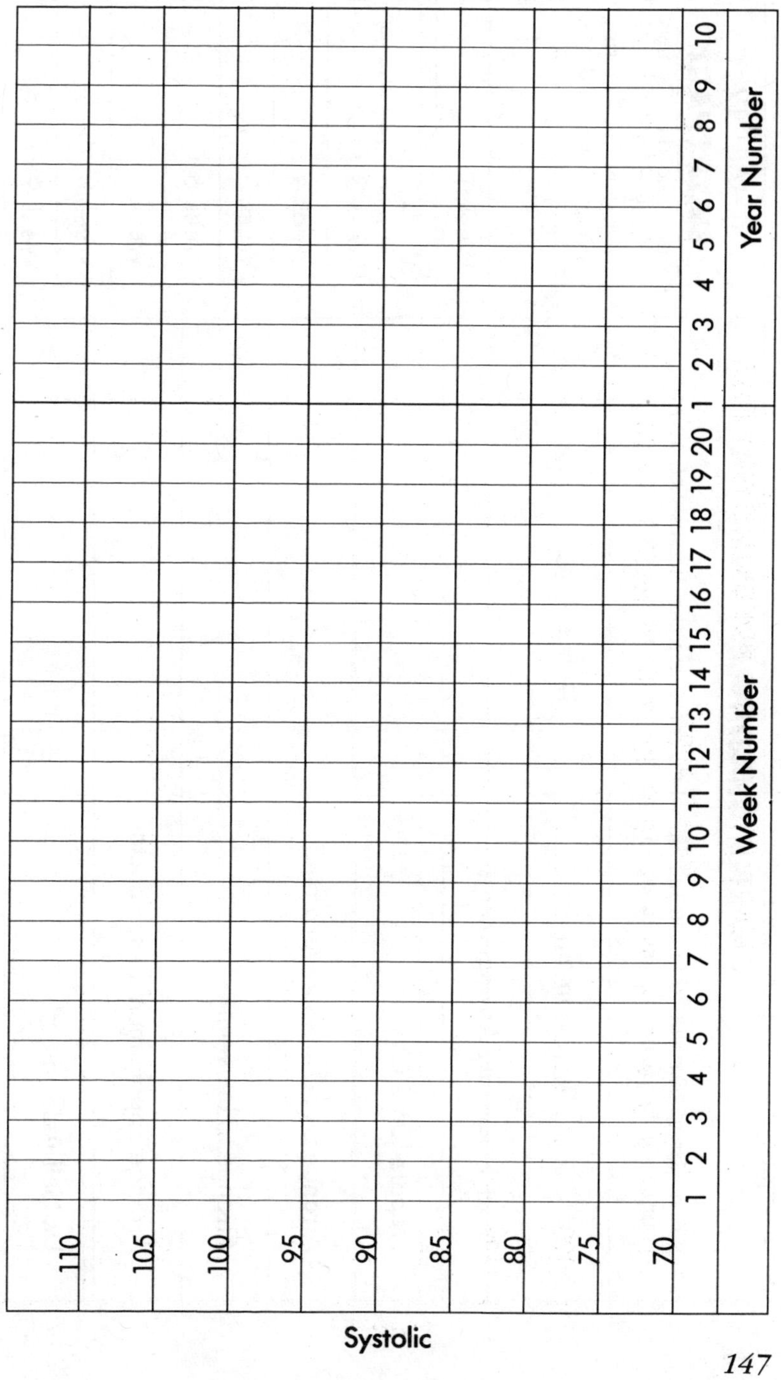
110
105
100
95
90
85
80
75
70
1 2 3 4 5 6 7 8 9 10 11 12 13 14 15 16 17 18 19 20
Week Number
1 2 3 4 5 6 7 8 9 10
Year Number
Systolic

CHART 11: **TIMETABLE**

When Harry asks you to make an appointment enter the details below. After completing the particular task enter a tick in the comments column.

Appointment	Date & Time	Comments
Read 'Necessary Arrangements'		
Prepare 'Date Chart'		
Arrange blood pressure recordings		
Arrange to be weighed		
Arrange appointment to see doctor		
Do 'Self Assessment'		

CHART 12: **DATE CHART**

Enter the date of next Sunday beside Week 1. Then continue entering the appropriate dates.

	Sunday Date
Week 1	
Week 2	
Week 3	
Week 4	
Week 5	
Week 6	
Week 7	
Week 8	
Week 9	

Work through 'Weigh Less'		
Highlight 'Good Eating Guidelines Check List'		
Work through 'Increase Activity'		
Complete 'My Exercise Program'		
Work through 'Not Too Much Grog'		
Work through 'Relax'		
Work through 'Ease Back On Salt'	Week 6	
Work through 'No More Smokes'	Week 10	
Read 'Harry's Healthy Hints'		

Week 10	
Week 11	
Week 12	
Week 13	
Week 14	
Week 15	
Week 16	
Week 17	
Week 18	
Week 19	
Week 20	

Optimist's Creed

Promise yourself

- to be strong so that nothing can disturb your peace of mind
- to talk health, happiness and prosperity to every person you meet
- to make all your friends feel good about themselves
- to look at the sunny side of everything and make your optimism come true
- to be just as enthusiastic about the success of others as you are about yourself
- to forget the mistakes of the past and press on to the greater achievements of the future
- to wear a cheerful countenance at all times and give every living creature you meet a smile
- to give so much time to the improvement of yourself that you have no time to criticise others
- to be too large for worry, too noble for anger, too strong for fear and too happy to permit the presence of trouble.

Anonymous

Whatever you do or dream you can — begin it
GOETHE

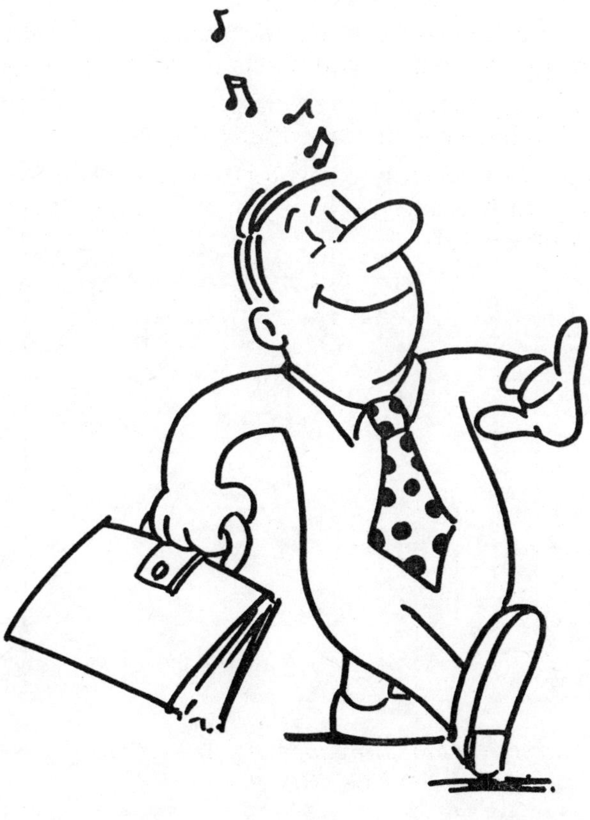